J. A. THOMPSON

The-Great-Burnout

Second edition

ISBN: 978-0-6457673-0-8

This book was professionally typeset on Reedsy.
Find out more at reedsy.com

Contents

Dedication

This book is dedicated to my late partner Brian, who is missed every day, he was my biggest fan and my biggest critic. We shared the love of books and he would have taken great pleasure editing this one for me... x

Introduction

B̲e master of your petty annoyances and conserve your energies for the big, worthwhile things.
It is not the mountain ahead that wears you out, it's the grain of sand in your shoe.
'Author-Robert Service'

In 2021 I experienced Burnout, on reflection it had been building up gradually, over many years, and I did not recognise the warning signs. It became one of the most debilitating and life-changing things I have ever gone through. A few times, during my worst periods, I did not believe I would ever return to my old self.

At my lowest point, in a state of being unable to think and unable to move, I convinced myself I must have the start of a serious illness; motor neuron disease or maybe even leukemia...

I had worked the last fourteen years for a private medical company, in various management roles. At the time of my resignation, I was working as a Business and Operations manager in their chronic disease treatment division, managing clinics across Melbourne, Adelaide, and Perth. I had been in this position for just over three years.

I handed my notice in on a Monday afternoon, it was an impulse decision, however I had been quietly quitting in my head for at least two years prior to this.

It was an amazing feeling – like I had finally let go of this great weight pushing down on my shoulders. The stress, the responsibility, the burden of it all began to just disappear that day, like a palpable release of negative energy lightening the weight with every thought.

Unfortunately, by Wednesday of that week I had started to develop a 'bit of a cold', and by Friday I was ill with a severe chest infection (non-COVID).

I became so sick I could not get out of bed, no matter how many cold and flu tablets I took, I could not shake the symptoms. Eventually I just relented, stopped fighting and ended up being unable to work any more of my four weeks' resignation period. I had to leave my job without saying goodbye in person to any of my employees. What was even worse, I didn't have the energy to care. I spent the following three months in a catatonic state between my bed and the sofa. I did not care what my future held, or how I was going to pull myself around.

My mind was just a blur, I was too exhausted to even walk up the stairs. Bills went unpaid, and I neglected my self-care. For my whole life I had always made a point of showing up with my hair done and make-up on. Yet here I was with unkempt hair and a bare face, not even bothering to clean my teeth some mornings.

This book is the story of burnout and why so many people at this moment from all over the world are becoming burned out. It tells my personal journey through this condition, as well as others. I have gradually recovered from this experience with more insight into my body and mind.

Examining burnout with my newfound knowledge and experience, I can hopefully help others recognise and prevent this happening to them and assist managers to look at burnout differently.

I do not profess to be an expert on burnout and its effects on us, however through my experience, I have gained a personal insight and knowledge. I have also spoken to others who have suffered similar experiences.

During this time, I kept a journal of sorts close by, sporadically documenting how I felt. It was heartbreaking for me to read it when I started writing this book. I hope this book will help encourage you, your employees, colleagues, or relatives to seek help and self-care promptly if you feel you are suffering from burnout.

My burnout crept up slowly, sneaking into my work and infiltrating my home life, as they both became increasingly stressful at the same time. This was exacerbated eventually in February of 2020 by the personal trauma of my partner of seventeen years taking his own life. This was followed quickly in March 2020 by the global coronavirus pandemic and subsequent lock downs.

I am a registered nurse with many years experience working with chronic diseases caused by long-term inflammation such as Type 2 diabetes and cardiovascular disease. Before suffering burnout, I had never given much consideration to the causal long-term effects of burnout on these processes. Nor had I thought about the intricate connection that exists between the mind, body, and inflammation.

After three years of pandemic worry, change and stress across the workforce, burnout – which is known as the carers' disease – is now affecting blue-collar and white-collar workers alike in developed countries across the world like never before.

Human resource managers are now using phrases such as 'Quiet Quitting and the 'Great Resignation'. I know for sure that this is all being caused by 'The Great Burnout'.

If you have a colleague or relative you believe is showing signs of burnout, I urge you to mention this book to them. This is not a condition to be taken lightly; it can have major consequences for the body and the mind.

I honestly believe that identifying signs of this early can lead to better outcomes for yourself and the organisation you work for.

I am committed to launching this book in an audio book too, as in my own experience I was unable to read books for months due to brain fog, being an avid book reader, I took solace in audio books during this time.

Writing this book has given me amazing insight into my own lack of self-care at the time, as well as the reasons why we are driven into this subconscious self-harm. I have just about come out the other side of this condition now, and want to share my journey with you.

Prologue - I Just Want to Sit on the Beach

I t's Monday morning in the middle of January and everyone is returning to work after their Christmas break. I worked over the Christmas period: it had been a hectic year and the holidays gave me time to do some planning for the new financial year, to try and have a head start on preparing year-end appraisals for my staff.

After psyching myself up with two consecutive cups of coffee, I turn on my computer and reluctantly start scanning through a relentless stream of emails. I see one that has the words 'My Resignation' in the title line and my heart sinks.

I am starting to feel stressed at little things lately. Everything is becoming emotional; I am taking everything to heart. I always used to be level-headed nothing was too much trouble. I was now overreacting to trivial things, as though they were the end of the world. Once I was deep into this emotional state I had trouble snapping out of it and focusing again on things I needed to do.

I click on the email, which is from Karen, one of my key employees. She has been in my team for over ten years and has only just returned to work that morning from three weeks leave. I curse, surely her time off had given her enough time for rest and recuperation. I take a deep breath and call her into my office to find out why she is leaving, and what I can do to make her stay. I need her desperately to stay...

I try to swallow down the lump in my throat, which seems to be expanding by the minute, and ask her if there is anything I can do to make her change her mind. She answers me calmly, and clearly as though she has spent the weekend in front of the mirror practicing, determined that I will not talk her out of it, but with an honesty that resonates with me and stayed with me, like a little seed planted in the back of my consciousness...

"I'm so sorry" she says..."I have given this a lot of thought over the last few months, I must go. I have just taken three week leave and I am still so exhausted. I have nothing left to give, now all I want to do is just to go and sit on the beach..."

If you live in the northern hemisphere this probably sounds like a strange thing to say in mid-January. However, we live on the west coast of Australia on the Indian ocean and here January is the middle of summer, with average temperatures in the mid to high thirties.

This was going to be disastrous. Karen was a critical member of my already under resourced team – not to mention the extra workload for me recruiting someone to replace her!

I was aware she had been pulled in all directions, we were expanding quickly, and the pressure was growing. Just add a global pandemic to the mix and it had pushed all my team to the brink.

I feel my heart rate rising, Karen coordinates all our clinical governance and COVID policies; it will take months to recruit someone and bring them up to speed with this.

"OK, that's cool" I say. "We can work around that". I offer her three months off work to recover. She declines, saying it's not enough: she needs to completely switch off, she is running on empty, and she can't go on like this. Eventually, sadly, I accept her resignation.

Ironically at this time, I didn't even comprehend the idea of burnout, and it hadn't occurred to me that she was suffering from it.

I would hear those same phrases over and over as I interviewed people for my book. 'Running on empty', 'nothing left to give' 'nothing left in the tank' 'my batteries are flat'. I even used them myself as I resigned. It's a need to assert the fact that you are so much more than tired, more than exhausted. It's not just your body, it's your mind as well – you're broken...

Four weeks later, as she was departing the clinic on her last day, I wished her luck and congratulated her on having the courage and self-awareness to come to this decision. I confided in her that I also needed to go and sit on the beach.

I knew then that I needed to do something, my work had just become too much, and I didn't know how much longer I could carry on showing up.

Writing this book, I have come to discover that burnout levels in society are currently higher than ever recorded. Evidence is pointing to the fact that this Great Burnout is a dangerous by-product of the COVID 19 pandemic.

In this book I will discuss why this is the case, and why burnout has such far-reaching consequences not only on our personal long-term health, but also on the global economy.

Chapter One - My Realisation

"**M**y Friend...care for your psyche...know thyself, for once we know ourselves, we may learn how to care for ourselves" – **Socrates.**

I live in Perth, Western Australia, in my last job before burning out, my office was eight minutes' drive from the nearest beach. We have some of the most pristine coastline in the world on our doorstep, which ironically was one of the reasons I emigrated here from the north of England, when I was thirty. I opted for a life of sunshine and beaches; for the quality of life Perth offered, a 'work to play' lifestyle. Yet here I was, burned-out and not having the time or strength to enjoy my surroundings – or my life, for that matter.

My colleague's resignation was a wake-up call. I had lost my direction. I was living in a city that holds the title of the sunniest state in the world and is continuously classed as one of the top ten most livable cities in the world, yet here I was spending my weekends lying on the sofa watching junk on TV.

I no longer had the desire or the energy to do anything other than try to get ready to show my face at work on a Monday morning again.

My load was getting heavier. I used to relish travel and be a social butterfly. A friend's father once described me as effervescent; I oozed energy and happiness. I now only savored staying at home, where I could

9

be in my quiet zone. I did not desire to speak or even listen to anyone, and I just wanted to go to bed early. These were all signs (although I did not know it at the time) of my precipitating burnout.

I know not everyone cares for the beach, or sunshine for that matter; however, we all have dreams of where our happy place is.

Have a think about where your happy place would be: where do you aspire to be in future? Would you want to go to the mountains, a picturesque country village, a cabin somewhere in the snow, where you can free ski every day? A country farmhouse where you can spend your days walking your dog through the hills, or fishing on the lakes?

What are your goals, and why are you working so hard?

Did you have dreams of where you were going with your life when you were younger? Are you still on that track, or have you strayed from that road and lost your way?

Have you reached the pinnacle of your career and are no longer feeling the love of life? Have your lines blurred between your work and home lives? Have you forgotten what is important along the way? I did ...

In my experience now, we need to keep a regular check on *why* we work and where we want to go. We all need money, and we all aspire to be successful. Money gives us means to do what we want to do. However, it does not bring happiness, and we need to keep reminding ourselves of this every now and again.

I loved my job. It became my life, and my employees became like my family. I became so consumed in my work that over the years I slowly began putting every other aspect of my life in second place. My partner, my family and friends, my health, and my well being. I became so consumed in my career that it morphed into my lifestyle.

Flying off to Sydney on a Sunday to be ready for a Monday morning meeting, then spending my Friday evenings in the airline lounge drinking wine on my way home – were the norm. I was sharing my calendar with my partner so he could keep track of what flights and what state I was working in, and when I would be coming home.

I was going so fast, but in my head, I really thought I was still managing to juggle all the balls in my life successfully. I thought I had it all – however really I was slowly drowning... and my world was falling in around me.

The years were just passing by quickly; my plate was constantly full, going from forecast to budget to end of fiscal year. Nothing was quite in control, everything was just pushing that bit further out of reach: bigger budgets to achieve, key performance indicators and efficiencies to meet.

I would work and work and then I would get a cold or flu and I just could not shake it. I would crash for a few weeks, apologising to everyone for letting them down, and then come back to work and hit the ground running again.

I always had an open-door policy in my office, employees were allowed to just to come in anytime and chat if the door was open, if it was closed they knew I was busy and this is how I liked it. I liked to know my employees personally, and this meant they were always happy to tell me what was happening at the coal face. This started to change, I would close my door and just work, I started avoiding the chats. Eventually I would prefer to work from home and was increasingly withdrawing from my team.

In the last 12 months, customers started to joke about me never answering my phone. I would just smile. What they did not realize was that I couldn't bear the sound of an incoming call any more–all the ringing and pinging. I was even reluctant to retrieve my voicemails in the end, as I knew it could be another fire to put out.

My daughter once noted that every time my phone rang, I would pull a face and curse. I couldn't even stand hearing my ringtone as my phone rang so often – I would eventually just leave it on silent permanently. To this day I still cringe on hearing the sound of the infamous Apple ringtone on other people's phones.

Researchers have described burnout as a chronic emotional, interpersonal stress. Employees suffer with overwhelming emotional exhaustion, feelings of cynicism and a lack of accomplishment. With retrospect I can now recognise that I was feeling all of these things a long time before I eventually crashed.

My own perception of what burnout looked like was just low energy: exhausted people needing a rest, as if they did not have the resilience to stay at this level. I believed that high-energy people like me did not burnout.

Having now just emerged to the surface after suffering from this debilitating condition, I would like to share with you my journey through burnout and to give you insight into the warning signs. Hopefully, this will assist you to recognise the signs of burnout and prevent either yourself, your employees, friends, or family from falling down this deep hole.

Saying I have come out of the other side would be optimistic. It's better to say I have changed. I can still feel it, and at the time of writing this I have not yet started another full-time job.

Burnout has been written about for years in different forms. In the 1960s it was called the 'carers' illness'. Doctors, nurses and caregivers alike were noted as suffering from idiopathic emotional and physical exhaustion that had no real diagnosis or name.

In recent years it has sometimes been referred to as adrenal fatigue, although this is not a medical term. Anne Kearns (PhD) states on the Mayo clinic website: "Adrenal Fatigue is not an accepted medical diagnosis. It is a lay term applied to a collection of nonspecific symptoms, such as body aches, fatigue, nervousness, sleep disturbances and digestive problems." Kearns goes on to say that proponents of the adrenal fatigue diagnosis claim this is a mild form of adrenal insufficiency (which IS a medical diagnosis) caused by stress.

Over the years work colleagues around me had used the term 'burnout' as a throw away comment (or so I thought). They felt burnt out or said things like "do not work for that company they burn their staff out". Yet here in 2023 we are seeing increasing population of people from all professions resigning due to burnout.

The Great Resignation is taking place around us, and companies are struggling to replenish staff. After burning out myself in 2021, I believe it is not 'The Great Resignation' we are seeing, but 'The Great Burnout'.

Masses of people have experienced great stress and uncertainty during this time within their work environment and their personal lives, uncertainty, and insecurity, which alone raises stress levels.

The Pandemic

Let us take a small step back to mid-January 2020. A zoonotic virus has spread across the Earth at an unheard of speed. The first doctor in Wuhan to alert the world on social media of this virus—and what was happening there—dies from it, followed over the next 12 months by thousands of nurses, doctors, and paramedics worldwide.

Nursing home residents, carers and taxi drivers all fall victim to this indiscriminate virus. The old and vulnerable, front line workers, friends, and family members were all taken. No-one knows anything about it, or how to stop it, other than isolation.

Governments worldwide grapple between locking down countries and financial security. Insecurity overcomes us all, and we suddenly face our mortality and that of our elderly and vulnerable relatives.

Meanwhile the world is trying to function. Stock markets have crashed, and food is visibly short on supermarket shelves due to panic buying and supply chain problems. We need to keep the workforce going, and there is an unpredictability to the world that we have never experienced before.

Social media sites are on fire. Fake news is more prevalent than ever, as everyone suddenly had an opinion on everything COVID-19

The way we worked changed overnight as lock downs started to be enforced across the world. By the end of March 2020 most countries had brought in restrictions and the way we worked and lived had changed.

Airplanes had grounded and socialisation in large groups was no longer allowed. The stresses of life elevated across every country in the world. People tried desperately to get home to families overseas before lock downs commenced.

Cruise ships sailed aimlessly from port to port unable to dock, whilst people were sick and dying on board. Others were locked down in their apartment buildings for weeks, socially isolated, while their relatives died alone and had funerals attended by few people, if they were lucky.

Companies adjusted to a 'new normal' to try to keep the world moving. Manufacturers of personal protective equipment (PPE), ventilators, and other medical equipment go into overdrive to keep front line workers protected.

Phrases such as social distancing, underlying medical conditions and close contacts became widely used.

Medical professionals grappled to find the best new treatment protocols to deal with the sick and dying. Scientists raced to find viable testing kits and vaccines, while health professionals worked on developing new directives of care for this new disease.

We were grounded! New computers were ordered for employee's homes, and IT specialists worked all hours to set up millions of employees up in their home offices or kitchen tables to keep the world running.

We have become accustomed now to seeing news presenters in their own homes, and repeats of TV soaps as they were no longer filming new episodes. Schools closed, and essential workers suddenly had to think about childcare and elderly care as well as doing their day-to-day work.

Companies were left with skeleton staff as people became close contacts. People resigned and left out of fear. Then, as weeks turned into months and months turned into years, came The Great Resignation. Why?

By 2021 professionals who had never previously experienced burn out, were suddenly suffering this debilitating exhaustion. Teachers, bankers, IT professionals were also becoming increasingly susceptible.

Start and end times at work suddenly became blurred, as employees tried to 'muck in' so we could keep things functioning. We became overwhelmed by the early-morning and late-night Zoom calls that had now become the norm.

As we were isolating, 24-hour news stations had our undivided attention, reporting daily death tolls and infection rates. We were no longer just watching a disaster unfolding in a foreign country; we were all in this together across the world. We were all feeling insecurity and worry for ourselves and our families.

Queuing for PCR tests and vaccinations became part of life. So, ultimately, did arguing with friends and acquaintances about how the pandemic was being managed. Overnight the general public became both politicians and epidemiologists, and had expert opinions on everything to do with COVID-19.

Meanwhile millions of people lost relatives and friends who had succumbed to this illness, or suffered from the lack of medical care due to overwhelmed health systems. Most of us were hurting or overwhelmed by the information overload we were receiving. By 2021 there were more mentally exhausted people in the workforce than ever before.

Non-front line workers spent months working from home, isolated from their colleagues, meaning no-one was picking up the well being and mental health of these employees.

Managers were – and still are in some places– managing their staff remotely with their only contact being through video calls. How can you really get to know employees properly this way, and pick up on signals of distress and discontent?

High-energy people in general, can manage high workloads (within reason), and can even thrive on them for set periods of time, if it creates success, recognition, and reward. Unfortunately, by adding in extra confusion and stress to the mix (in terms of work or personal life), the tipping point gets ever closer.

I loved my job, I loved the people I worked with and always thought I would be there until I retired. The challenges were great, the business model was great, and to top it all off, for all I was super busy, I had autonomy.

Things changed around three years before I left, when there was a big management shakeup at director level. I suddenly felt insignificant. I had won and managed the biggest contract the company had ever had in Australia – regrettably no-one seemed to know this or recognize what this meant anymore. My opinions and contribution were ignored, and I started to become cynical about the company's direction.

Was the cynicism that comes with burnout making me over-sensitive? Retrospectively my cynicism was justified; sadly, my frustration and reaction to this were signs that I was at the start of my burnout journey.

Around this same time my partner started suffering from severe anxiety and depression which was starting to both worry me and distract me as I tried to get him the care he needed. I had neither experience or understanding of dealing with these issues.

My daughter gave birth to my first grandson, and I remember sitting in a meeting receiving texts of how she was progressing, eventually excusing myself, so I could be with her when she had the baby. To top it off my son was in a car accident that left him in a wheelchair with a broken back and two broken legs. I tried to keep calm and just continue.

My partner devastatingly took his own life in February 2020, I was heartbroken and guilt ridden that I was unable to prevent this. My mother came from the UK to give me support and I stayed off work for three weeks.

Unfortunately, due to the start of the pandemic lockdowns, my mother had to hurry back to the UK while she could still get out and so I decided to distract myself, I should return to work.

I threw myself totally into my work, and by the time 2021 arrived, my partner's clothes were still on his side of the wardrobe, and his ashes were still in the plastic crematorium container, sleeping on his side of the bed next to me.

I was feeling exhausted, I needed some time out...

In Australia, if it is part of your employment contract, you are entitled to long service leave after ten years of permanent employment. This tends to be around twelve weeks paid leave and my long service leave was now four years overdue.

I was becoming desperate to take this time off, but like a lot of people, I was thinking what would I do with all this time off and nowhere to go! West Australian borders were still closed so if I holidayed it was within the state and we were so under-resourced that I knew that if I asked to take it, it would not be approved.

Taking time off sick was out of the question. I thought I would appear weak in front of my colleagues, and physically I was OK. Sort of...

I was indecisive and could not trust my own decision-making skills anymore. I was frightened that if I resigned, I would regret it. So, I continued...

As a type A personality, a high achiever and an adrenaline junkie, I thrived on challenges and prided myself on this. So was I changing or just getting old? Why was I feeling this overwhelming need to retreat?

After Karen left in February 2021 to go and sit on the beach, I carried on – however that seed was well and truly planted and was niggling away at me. I needed to go and sit on the beach every day, that would heal me...

I made up my mind, I now had a plan, I would hand in my resignation, December of that year, it was now May. Ironically I only lasted until August...

Chapter Two - The Motivation That Drives Us

"**W**onder is the beginning of Wisdom" – Socrates

To examine burnout fully we must first look at our motivation. If we were not driven or motivated, we wouldn't burn out. In fact, we would not even want to work.

Motivation is the catalyst driving us to take all action in life and has allowed us to evolve as humans into a superior race in comparison to other species. All actions we take simple, or complex have a motivation behind them.

What makes us think we are superhuman and so important that we feel life in our workplace cannot survive without us? What gives us that motivation to put so much effort and energy into our work, is it to be successful for recognition.

What motivates you? Are our drivers of success also the reasons for our downfall, allowing ourselves to burn out?

We tell our children that they must work hard at school to become successful. How do we then define success? To achieve good exam results, go to university and find a profession that gives us financial security and respect?

Let us be honest: what is the first question you ask a person when you first meet them? What do you do for a living? What line of work are you in? Does this sound familiar? Even now, as I am half-way through a year of not working, I still at times find it uncomfortable to define myself and what I do to new people.

I do not believe there is anything wrong with job satisfaction and financial stability, its great to love your work and get paid to do what you love, however, a person's profession should not be there only measure of success. This can set children and young adults up for failure and under achievement.

John Lennon supposedly once said: *"When I was five years old my mother told me that happiness is the key to life. When I went to school, they asked me what I wanted to be when I grew up. I wrote down 'happy.' They told me I didn't understand the assignment. I told them they didn't understand life"*.

We strive for a better house, car, clothes, and gadgets. After every promotion we upgrade our lifestyle. Recently I caught up with my ex-boss who has now been retired for a few years. She was telling me how she had a whole wardrobe of expensive designer suits that she no longer needed, and a box full of designer scarves she used to just buy on a whim while traveling. Now she wears predominantly joggers, no jewelry or makeup, except when she is heading out socially – which, let's face it, has been a rarity for us all over the last few years. She feels like it has all just been a huge waste of money.

What drives us to this state of needing increasingly more, and not listening to our bodies giving us subtle hints about when to stop?

There is a well-known saying: no-one says on their deathbed that they wished they had spent more time at work. I believe that money gives us freedom, not happiness – so if we keep being slaves to money, we will never be happy.

Motivations has been described by some, as a carrot and a stick phenomenon. On one side we have the carrot being the goal, the things we strive for in our lives such as success, money and freedom.

On the other side we have the stick, which is fear, fear of what life holds if we do not do or achieve these things, whether it be money, success or freedom. It could be fear of poverty if your parents were poor, fear of not having the freedom to move somewhere different.

Maslow's Hierarchy of Needs

Searching for answers to what our motivations are, I immediately revisited Abraham Maslow's Hierarchy of Needs, which I originally became familiar with when training to be a nurse.

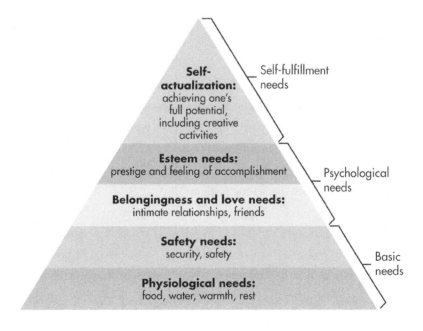

Maslow's Hierarchy of Needs (1943)

All individual priorities and needs start at the bottom of the pyramid and as each need is met, we are motivated to work our way up in order.

Self-Actualization is classed as a growth need not an essential need as the others and not everyone reaches this stage in their development.

According to Maslow we have five types of needs:

Physiological: These needs are the starting point for human motivation and are called the physiological drives. They include food, water and clothing, and anything that we need at a basic level to survive.

Safety: Security of oneself physically and mentality, security of one's employment, safety of one's environment, family, and health.

This is one aspect which has been challenged greatly by the pandemic, and it is one of the reasons why some of us kept going and could not give up the security of our jobs.

Love & Belonging: Friendship networks, family support, sexual intimacy, social acceptance of who we are and our individuality.

My comment earlier in the chapter on how we ask people what they do for a living, to define them into our acceptance criteria, does this contribute to all of Maslow's needs? Like Socrates the more I delve into this subject the more questions I ask.

Esteem: (self and from others.) Could this be why social media and the culture of instant gratification is so popular? Do our egos push us to our careers and money? Are our motivations becoming our downfall? I do not have the answers to this as everyone's case is different; **but**, I believe that these are major contributing factors to burnout.

Self-Actualisation: (Achieving one's individual potential) As shown in Maslow's pyramid, a person's basic needs must be met before self-actualisation can be achieved. This includes morality, creativity, problem solving, and acceptance of facts.

Is this what drives us, to fulfilling our needs? Not everyone manages to reach this level of self-actualization. Is the push to do so a contributing factor to burnout?

Recognition and Reward

When working in sales, I once remember pushing myself so hard to earn a monetary bonus. At some point I realised that the system was rigged against me, I could never achieve its full potential, at this point, I stopped trying.

In other words, if something is unachievable you lose energy and in fact become *demotivated.* This also applies if you feel that no-one is listening to you. Eventually you realise you are treading water, no one cares and so you give up.

On the other hand, working with achievable targets, and having the chance to gain recognition and reward, can motivate and energise you.

In 2001 I attended a pharmaceutical conference in Hawaii, we worked from 8am to 6pm every day, followed by adrenaline rush activities such as Harley Davidson rides down Waikiki beach, jet skiing, paragliding, waterparks etc.

At the conference close, we all felt energised despite five, non-stop, action-packed days and knowing we had long flights back to Australia. We were all happy, pumped and eager to start launching the new product on our return and we also knew the company was going to be recognising and rewarding us generously for this. We had been served our bonus plan as the finale' on the last day of the conference and were all excited to be making some extra cash.

I arrived back in Perth on a Sunday evening and I was out on my territory working first thing on the Monday morning. I was also motivated by the next exciting reward: a trip to a conference in Europe. I had not seen my family in the UK for over three years, and this could give me the opportunity to do so, I pushed on with determination and won this prize.

My point being, your body can cope with high-energy work for short periods if it has an end date and you have recognition and reward for what you are doing. If no-one is listening to you or caring for you, if you are having workloads pushed on to you with no sign of a reprieve, you lose energy, long-term this becomes lethargy. Add to this some stress that has no end date and we have lift-off: you are burning out!

Have you ever felt elated about something and then excitedly shared your information with someone who wasn't at all interested, or was critical? Did you feel deflated? Disappointment? Exhausted?

Imagine feeling this level of deflation every day? Having to psych yourself up to go into the office to face negativity, an unrelenting workload and not being able to see any light at the end of the tunnel. Working full time is hard enough without having to use all this extra energy on negative stress.

Creativity

"Creativity is just intelligence having fun"- **Albert Einstein**

Creativity is left brain activity and working for public listed companies, with large budgets, crunching numbers on endless spreadsheets, is right brain activity.

If you are left brain dominant, which I believe I am, this overload tends to stifle your creative side. You need space and time to think and develop creative thoughts.

This is one of the reasons why Google and other Silicon Valley companies create chilled spaces for their employees, to empty their minds and induce creativity.

I like to think my creative mind is one of my strengths. I was known to my colleagues as an 'ideas' person; however, as my workload grew, I noticed my creativity was soon crowded out with menial tasks and 'fires to fight' which filled my days. This became a noticeable thing to me and troubling. I would keep pushing it to the back of my mind thinking that as soon as I had some quiet time it would return, of course eventually there was no quiet time, and my creative potential was lost for many years.

Companies must understand that if they want growth and to culti-vate innovative ideas to increase productivity, over burdening their employees will prevent this and deplete energy. This can eventually mean some companies are left behind when change happens in their business landscape as they struggle to see the wood for the trees. For example Kodak when digitalisation came or Blockbuster turning down the opportunity of purchasing Netflix.

Arduous work without any engagement and keeping staff in the dark to the company's strategic plan, kills motivation and creativity. Staff want to be part of innovative ideas and to grow with the company, if they are not heard and left to just work hard, without inclusiveness, they will leave moving on to somewhere they will feel they are wanted and belong or they will stay and burn out.

In later years most of my ideas tended to occur either in a car or on a plane, this was due to me, not receiving or answering texts, phone calls or emails, I had room for thought.

When the pandemic arrived in 2020, I stopped travelling. Suddenly I was always available. My work–life balance suffered: my diary became public to the company and was available for anyone to put in meeting requests as they wished.

There was no longer travel time in my calendar so the meetings would be back to back and I would spend entire days on Zoom or Microsoft office calls, this became the new norm, not only for myself but for many people around the world...

Chapter Three - Recognising the Signs of Burnout

"**B**eware of the Barrenness of a busy life"- **Socrates**

I cannot stress enough that burnout is a gradual process. It is not a case of "Phew, I've been crazy busy the last few weeks, I must have burn out". That would just be fatigue or physical exhaustion, and if you are fit and healthy, you should be able to bounce back from this, with a few days of rest.

It's a chronic, build up over time, due to living with elevated levels of the stress hormone cortisol in your bloodstream.

Burnout has been written about in different forms since the seventies, The studies have been vague, due to differing symptoms and situations. As a result, no single diagnosis has ever given to it.

That was until 2019, when the World Health Organization (WHO) officially recognized burnout as a medical diagnosis.

WHO has defined burnout in their International Classification of Diseases handbook (ICD-11): *Burnout is a syndrome conceptualized as resulting from chronic workplace stress that has not been successfully managed and is categorized in 3 dimensions:*

1. *Feelings of energy depletion*

2. *Increased mental distance from one's job or feelings of negativism or cynicism related to one's job.*

3. *Reduced professional efficacy.*

It goes on to state Burnout is officially a chronic workplace phenomena in the occupational context and should not be applied to describe experiences in other areas of life...

Historically, burnout has never been recognised as an illness or a condition and for all WHO have fallen short by just recognizing burnout as a syndrome, it's a starting point and we know more research needs to be done in this area to gain a better understanding and recognition.

I must add at this point, my view is, burnout is NOT always caused by work, there can be other external contributing factors that trigger burnout on their own.

Carers looking after family members with complex, chronic diseases such as Multiple Sclerosis or Alzheimer disease, having to perform daily treatments for their loved ones such as home dialysis, can suffer from burn out. These conditions long term put both psychological and physical stress on the carers with no end date, little recognition, and exhaustion. These carers are also probably suffering with guilt and social isolation, charity organisations recognise this burnout and specifically cater for these people with respite care, as do a lot of health services to ease this burnout.

The WHO guidelines definition for burnout does not make allowances for these people in their classification. I look forward to seeing further recognition of burnout by the World Health Organization as a medical condition in near future years.

13 Early Signs of Burnout

Vanessa Loder, wrote an article for Forbes in 2015 giving what she believes are the 13 early signs of burnout:

1.High levels of stress and anxiety - Feeling frequently on the edge, with adrenaline constantly coursing through your body.

2.Lack of engagement - You do not feel motivated to work. Difficulty to focus or exhibiting a short attention span.

3.Increased cynicism – Feelings of resentment or disconnection. Feeling negative and frustrated.

Adding in some of my own thoughts in here, as I can personally relate to them: The cynicism comes from the fact that you have been asking for help for so long and it is falling on deaf ears or so you perceive (whether real or unreal) that the management above you does not care. You feel undervalued and unheard.

4.Distracted eating- You eat your meals in front of a computer or TV or while on the go (in the car or standing up).

5.Not getting enough sleep – Less than seven hours per night.

6.Low energy and exhaustion – Not just sleepy, but emotionally and mentally fatigued. No matter how much sleep you have, you cannot shake the feeling of being exhausted.

7.Never enough time – Feeling as though you are always in a hurry, constant deadlines to meet. Always chasing your tail. In fact, you're productivity has dropped due to their exhaustion and you are struggling to keep on top of things.

For myself, this led to procrastination, constantly putting off those tasks that needed due diligence, such as numbers on spreadsheets or proof reading etc.

8.Excessive worry and self-criticism – Your mind cycles through the same worry filled thoughts repeatedly and you can't seem to stop them. A critical voice in your head is telling you to constantly work harder.

In my own experience; Due to my exhaustion, I was constantly coming down on myself thinking I was lazy. If a person feels like they have no control over their work, either due to a bad manager or a chronic high-pressure environment, no recognition or support, this can contribute to these feelings.

9.Physical illness – Initially subtle headaches, colds, and a weak immune system in general.

My own view is; If you are experiencing a weak immune system, this is not an early sign but a sign your body has been under continuous stress for extended periods of time and your immune system is now under extreme pressure due to this.

I would also add on to this in the early stages of burnout, heartburn, indigestion and bowel problems, either bouts of diarrhoea or constipation can often be experienced as very early symptoms of burnout as your digestive system responds to the stress hormones you are releasing causing over production of acid in your stomach and increased peristalsis (natural movement of the intestine).

Any inflammatory conditions you suffer from can flare up, such as dermatitis, psoriasis, Crohn's disease, rheumatoid arthritis. Viruses also start to sneak in when your immune system is depleted such as cold sores (herpes simplex) Shingles (Herpes Zoster) and you can become more susceptible to complications of viruses such as Guillain-Barre' syndrome (complication of the influenza virus).

10.Numb feelings- Increase in addictive behavior. Initially, this can show up as an excessive dependence of caffeine and or sugar to boost energy when feeling low, eventually leading on to dependencies on drugs, alcohol, comfort foods. Even watching more TV than usual can be a sign you are using coping mechanisms to avoid acknowledging how you really feel.

11.Inefficacy- Diminished personal accomplishment, a perceived decline in competence or productivity and expending energy at work without seeing any results. You are now treading water at this stage and are becoming ineffective.

12.No Breaks- You work through your day without taking any breaks. Not getting up from your workspace at least once an hour, to have a drink and stretching your legs can really put unnecessary stress on your body. Dehydration can make you feel worse. You cannot remember the last time you had a holiday where you just relaxed and did nothing. Weekly rituals – You have not made time for a rejuvenating activity in the last week for yourself.

13.Not enough Exercise- You are not making time to exercise or move your body as you would like.

Myself for 13, I will add on that due to the high cortisol (stress hormones) you tend to gain more weight, eat less healthy foods, and drink less water which in turn makes you become fatigued and reluctant to exercise. Ironically exercise and hydration are the two thing that can help 'blow off 'these stress hormones. Sadly, the things you least want to do are the things that can help you keep this under control in the beginning.

You will see different manifestations of these symptoms appearing in different people's accounts throughout this book, including my own account and if you do have burn out or know someone with it will recognise these signs in yourself.

My Own Burnout Symptoms

Interestingly, reflecting on all the symptoms on the previous pages of burnout and relating to them all now, and a few more! I ask myself why I did not worry about the way I was feeling and try to fix the situation earlier.

In answer to this after much reflection, I have to say firstly it became 'the norm', it was how I felt and I believed, eventually, when I slowed down, I would be fine again. The other reason I believe is, that I did not really know about burnout and what actually happened to you physically and mentally. If someone had said to me, if you keep going you will crash and I knew what that crash looked like. I may have listened and reacted sooner or differently.

I have written this book to make people aware and be frightened if they are experiencing these symptoms.

In my own role, despite feeling exhausted and oblivious to these symptoms in a way, although struggling, I carried on. I was frustrated with the company and was cynical to everything that was being laid out on the agenda. I was no longer enjoying coming to work. In my head I was imagining resigning, but was worried about losing my financial security and my house (Maslow's hierarchy of needs).

I started looking for other jobs, but 'couldn't be bothered' to apply for anything, and was too tired even to update my resume'.

I was procrastinating increasingly, leaving most of my tasks for Friday, which made me even more stressed as the week went on and having to work late on a Friday night to finish off. I would wake up around 3 or 4am and sometimes come downstairs and watch TV for an hour and then go back to bed. Other times if I woke at 4am I would think it was acceptable to get up and work.

Consuming increased amounts of coffee became the norm, unsuccessfully trying to bring myself back up with energy that was not there, boosting this with sugary snacks to try to get the same effect. Obviously with my high cortisol levels my metabolism was sluggish and I was putting on weight, which was then, contributing to my overall general feelings of lethargy.

I bought a Fitbit and started to monitor my sleep patterns which showed me I was consistently between 5 and 6.5 hours per night with the occasional 8 hour on a weekend. I would see my heart rate raise above one hundred beats per minute whilst I was sleeping at times. With my exercise, I tried to do at least 10,000 steps a day. Regrettably, some days I was finishing work and had only done 3,000, I did not have the energy to go out and move after work to boost this.

I became unsociable at work and couldn't face any conflict. Staff noticed I was disappearing from the front line more and more. I was able to work from home and just sit at my computer all day and not have contact with the outside world, except via email.

With hindsight I was no good to anyone during this period, and was doing a disservice to myself, my team and my employer as well.

Due to having all new managers at executive level and the borders between states closed, no-one knew me or had a baseline for my work, so no-one would have been able to recognize the change in my behavior.

If you are reading this and relate to it, please seek help, I believe the longer you leave this untreated, the harder it becomes to make rational decisions and the harder you crash. During the latter period, I was trying to take the odd days off to recharge; this was not enough to allow me to switch off. Even taking a week off at this stage is not doing anything as it tends to take the first three days of your holiday to start to winding down, so taking just one week or even two does not work.

The last time I remember being totally refreshed from a holiday was in 2016, I went on a holiday to Europe for a month including a Mediterranean cruise and remember coming back to work totally refreshed. Time completely away from my phone and laptop really helped me to recharge, I felt amazing on my return to work and believe people should do this for their own personal care and maybe if I had been able to do this annually it would have been enough.

The culture of the business I was working in was that you called people on their days off, after hours and even on holidays. We ran a patient focused business, the patients had to come first. With reflection, I do actually believe if a few more processes had been fixed 'up stream' in the supply chain area, the stress levels would have been less downstream at the customer facing level, which could have alleviated this.

There was also an expectation, not only across my area of work but with others I worked with externally that emails would be responded to immediately. This is not an acceptable expectation and I have had multiple phone calls from customers complaining they sent an email to me an hour ago and they have not had a response yet.

Has having emails on phones given work colleagues and customers more access to you and raised expectations for your responses to them? Are these also becoming a distraction for us to focus in the now?

Eventually I knew I needed a plan, an end date, I was only just tolerating my work. My plan was, I would give four weeks' notice in December of that year to finish after Christmas. I could then use my long service leave and accumulated holidays to take the rest of summer and the financial year off. I had three years of tax I hadn't submitted so knew I had some money that would be coming back from that also. This would enable me to be ready for a fresh new job at the beginning of the new fiscal year in July.

Once I gave myself this date, I felt a bit more in control however it was still only July and I knew I had another six months to work. I think at this point I was really starting to struggle; I just needed to sit tight and start planning my handover plan. I was pushing myself over the finish line with concrete boots on.

One Monday in early August, I was interviewing a staff member for an internal role, which would support me in my role (which I had been requesting for over twelve months). During the interview, the candidate told me how excited and energized she was feeling, and how this role was ideal for her career pathway.

At this point, I suddenly felt drained, uninspired and I realised I no longer had a clear career pathway myself. I was not energised, and this was probably one of the reasons why I no longer knew where I was heading and had no direction or focus. This was not me: I was positive and passionate by nature; I did not recognise myself anymore.

I had this sudden urge come over me, I had to go... NOW!

I came out of that interview gasping for air as though I was rising to the top of the water after being under it too long, I was suffocating and had to get out of there. I just wanted to leave work, go home never to return.

Instead, I went into my office, closed the door and wrote out my notice, I then pressed the send button. I wasn't totally sure how I was going to manage financially, and I really was past the stage of caring at this point.

There was a feeling of immediate relief once I had spoken to my boss, who incidentally said it was a great shock. I felt like I had a vice removed from my chest: I was going to be free.

By Wednesday of that week I had developed a bit of a sniffle so worked from home. But by Friday I was in bed with a full-blown chest infection. I had COVID symptoms, including losing my taste and smell, but tested negative twice. Due to this infection I never returned to the office...

I had crashed and burned.

I spent most of my first three months off work in a catatonic state between the sofa and the bed, unable to look at a computer or talk on a phone. I had no concentration and my head felt like it was full of cotton wool. I did not empty my work bag for three months. I felt like I was never going to be my old self again. I also thought I was going to have to buy a single-storey house as whenever I had to walk upstairs, I became physically exhausted and had to lie down on my bed to recover.

I knew I wanted to write this story, although I felt like I would never have the energy to do so. I had to keep a to-do list on my kitchen counter of the menial things I needed to do in my life, these menial things became like mountains to climb daily. I would have to psych myself up on a morning to do them, even if it was just a simple phone call to make, it was an effort, I just set myself a target of doing one thing a day.

I had purchased a new laptop when I knew I was leaving my job, but could not even face opening it to set it up. It took me seven months to open it and install Windows. I only used my phone reluctantly for emails. I had completely shut down. I did start to keep a bit of a diary – well, a sporadic mind dump really, of how I had been feeling. Some (unedited) snippets are below.

- Spending Saturdays on the sofa watching junk TV trying to recharge.
- Impatience with processes, everything is taking too long to happen.
- Falling asleep as soon as my head hit the pillow.
- Waking up early, stressed
- Procrastination
- Struggling to open my laptop. (Avoidance)
- Disinterested in socialising, mixing, or meeting with friends.

· Struggling to make any plans.

· Cringing when my phone rings; keeping it on silent as it triggers me.

· Wanting to buy a caravan and travel around Australia with my dogs only!

· Constantly craving peace and quiet.

· Feeling weak and lethargic at the slightest exertion.

· Difficulty making decisions.

· Swallowing copious amounts of vitamins to try and give me energy.

· More susceptible to infections and taking longer to recover.

· Constantly resigning in my head.

· Constant negativity to anything work related.

Is anyone out there relating to any of this? Do you have any symptoms of your own to add?

If you are feeling any of the above, please stop now and start making plans to at least have a month's break from work to recharge. If not, you will not even have the energy or concentration to even read this book in a few months' time.

Here are some excerpts from my diary over the first few weeks after I left work.

6 September 2021

Feeling guilty about being too sick to finish off everything at work however as soon as I realised I.T. had locked me out of the company system, it was a relief and I have let go.

Still too exhausted to walk.

10 September 2021

Went to Kmart tonight for a look out! Felt exhausted and breaking out in a sweat. Went to bed at nine and fell asleep as soon as my head hit the pillow.

Week three of not working

I've been approached by a recruitment agent about a General Managers role, they want me to fill out a statement of experience, procrastination kicked in and couldn't face opening my PC. I will decline.

With hindsight I would not have been doing myself or a new employee a favour jumping into a position at that stage.

Week four of not working

- *Weight gain +++*
- *Lethargic*
- *Weather is warming up, can't even face my to do list.*

This is all so painful for me to read and look back on now.

At this point you may be asking why I did not go to my employer and ask for time off from instead of leaving my job?

The previous year, I had asked my manager for four weeks leave during a major family crisis. He told me I could only have two weeks. I could not possibly go back to him again and be told the same thing – or even worse, be accused of not coping with my job.

I also did not feel it was fair or appropriate that during the pandemic, when everyone was working beyond their limits, I could expect to be granted a year off, which is what I knew I would need to recover. I think in hindsight I also knew it was time for me to move on.

Working in health management for a private expanding medical company, I was in the middle of some new clinic fit outs and was also managing a high value government contract when COVID 19 came. The pressure in my job was already immense, I was managing three

Australian states, so dealing with three public health systems, which all had unique needs and requirements to adhere to.

The state of Victoria was already feeling the effects of the pandemic badly, and we were having to keep constantly updated with the Victorian state health system. All three states were on different time zones so my days could start at 5am due to the three hour time difference. To say the pandemic brought in a significant layer of complexity and stress was an understatement.

Examining some other occupations other than in the medical field, who were feeling the stress during the pandemic, I have listed below some examples. I am sure you have your own stories to tell about the extra workload and stress this put on an already lean workforce.

- **IT-** suddenly had a huge workload increase trying to supply and connect hundreds of workers in their own homes and running help lines to keep the staff functioning.
- **Supply Chain-** sickness across all areas of staff, lock downs in China and stock backups in ports both locally and internationally.
- **Supermarket staff-** suddenly became the target of the public, working long hours with the risk of being exposed to the virus as well as having to police customers, who were panic buying and not wearing their masks.
- **Politicians-**having to enforce lock downs and face criticism daily at news updates.

Burnout vs PTSD

Dr. Geri Puleo, in her TEDx presentation compares the similarities of the symptoms of burnout with those of Post-Traumatic Stress disorder (PTSD) and goes as far as to say she believes burnout could be a form of PTSD.

Although PTSD is commonly associated with soldiers in war-time experiences, Puleo felt her participants experiences due to poorly led organisations, created the same reactions.

PTSD Characterisations also experienced by Burnout sufferers

- Exposure to a traumatic event OR extreme stressor
- Respond with fear, hopelessness, or horror.
- Sleep disturbances and nightmares
- Depression, withdrawal
- Frequent mood changes, generalised irritability
- Avoid activities that promote recall of traumatic events.

After reading this, reflecting back to myself, being unable to listen to my iPhone ringtone without cringing with a counsellor, who believed it was a sign of PTSD.

Sue's Burnout - Financial Sector:

Sue has worked as an executive manager in the financial sector for over ten years and has asked to remain anonymous. She believes working in a male dominant environment such as finance she has had to work hard to gain her position and gain respect. She believes her burnout will be perceived as a weakness.

The first thing she tells me is that this is not just about the work, and this has not just happened since 2020. She lost her husband to cancer ten years ago and has been bringing up two teenage children on her own and working full-time in Sydney's Central Business District, which is over an hour away by train from her home.

Her children are now at university and pre-pandemic she commuted her journey to work each way, listening to her music and podcasts. Looking back, she thinks unintentionally her train ride was maybe her way of psyching herself up for her workday, leaving her home life behind and for winding down each day on her way home after work.

Sue has always worked long days, which was the norm in her profession and was not a problem. She's a perfectionist by her own admission and is happy to work hard just to get the job done. She works in a male dominated area and feels like she has always had to prove herself working that extra bit harder to gain recognition and promotions. She is successful, intelligent, and humble on all fronts.

In 2020 like so many other people her life changed. Suddenly in March

2020 Australia went into lock down and we all had to work differently. Without going into the complexities of her work, the financial volatility and instability started to cause huge stresses to her work life.

During lock down, she was happy to leave her commute behind and was even happy to add those two hours travel time on to her workday. Like many of us over this time she was working long hours in her home, going from back-to-back video meetings all day long from early mornings to late at night.

We discussed the whole Microsoft ' Teams' meeting scenario, (Video Conferencing) as this was one of my big stressors during lock down. She explained that pre-pandemic you walked into a meeting, and you could read the room, you knew body languages, you could position yourself on what was happening and respond accordingly.

She believed that on the Teams meetings, you could not pick up people's body language and no room reading was possible, which meant you felt like you had lost one of your senses, thus having to work harder to communicate your points of view. This in turn was making her and everyone else exhausted. This I thought was an interesting point and had never come across the analogy before.

Walking out after face-to-face meetings, she went on to explain, this had always been a time to debrief and discuss what had gone on in the meeting with her colleagues. This was now impossible especially as with back-to-back meetings there was no time to reflect, debrief or plan. It was just straight on to the next meeting.

On top of the instability in the financial market, she had a team to now manage remotely. This of course came with its own dynamics: one team member had family in Europe that were in a COVID epicenter, as well as team members trying to cope with no childcare.

She took on more work to shield her team from these eccentricities – and one of her own team members who left her job had her work passed over to her rather than filling the position. By her own admission she is not assertive enough and struggles to say no. She believed it was a short-term inconvenience and did it just to get the job done.

The international customers she deals with mean she can be in meetings from 10pm to 3am; she is then allowed to start work later the next day to compensate for this late night. During the pandemic she wanted to be there for her team, so continued to start early, even after those 3am finishes.

After the first lock down in 2020 finished, there was a bit of an interlude and life began to regain some of normality and she continued to work from home in a hybrid way. She confessed she had noticed she was having to dig a lot deeper for energy, despite this she continued to work on weekends to keep up.

Then in 2021 Sydney went into a second long lock down as the second wave of the virus hit. With this her stresses from before came back stronger. She had an employee stuck in an apartment block in Melbourne that was locked down and she was trying to keep her own staff's morale up.

She recalls one of her direct reports saying she never wanted to be like her and work so much...

She was trying to keep normality for her children who were also studying from home, however felt she was there physically but not mentally. One day her daughter said to her: "you no longer hear me".

During this lock down, working from home, she changed roles. This new position had its own whole new set of challenges and technical issues, and she felt like she fell back into her old behaviors from the previous lock down seven months before.

She noticed that if she went into the kitchen for anything or stopped for lunch, she would avoid her study and would walk the long way around to avoid her laptop. This laptop avoidance started to increase as time went on.

One morning she woke up and just could not get out of bed. Both physically and mentally she felt empty, and she literally felt she could no longer do her job. She called in sick and confided to her manager that she could not get up out of bed. He was understanding, and suggested she then booked some sessions of counseling with the Employee Assistance Program, who diagnosed her with burnout.

She took three weeks off work and rested, and then returned. Asking her if she experienced any symptoms leading up to the burnout, she said she hadn't really been thinking about it, it just happened. However when I explained some of my symptoms, she admitted she probably was getting annoyed a lot more often, and was always assuming a negative stance. She also confessed she was not as effective when she was exhausted.

I asked her how she was feeling now, and she said she was still exhausted but she was being careful not to fall back into her old behaviors. I was still quite concerned about her and didn't feel like she had given herself enough time to recover, so I asked her what her boss would say if she requested three months off work to recover properly. She admitted she had never thought about it, but her accumulated leave and long service leave were constantly being pushed back, so it probably wouldn't be approved.

Sue accepted she needed to manage herself and her self-care better and that being a perfectionist was not helping her exhaustion. When I asked her on reflection what she had learned from this experience, she said felt her own behaviors had caused this, so she was managing her time better now.

She stated she was no longer working weekends, however on further questioning admitted she wouldn't fully commit to herself not to work the weekend otherwise this added to her stressors, therefore, she would commit to having only a Saturday morning off. She would then check her emails on a Saturday afternoon and if they were clear she would have the rest of the weekend off.

I must admit when talking to Sue I became worried about her health and well being long term, so we did discuss oxidative stress and inflammation caused by the long term effects of stress hormones on the body and I advised her to go and see her GP for a checkup and blood tests – she said she thinks she is OK.

On reflection she says she recognizes her blind spots and to help her manage her time better she was blocking out fake meetings in her calendar, to allow for time to reflect and retain positivity.

In my opinion Sue could be vulnerable to a further severe episodes of residual burnout down the line if any stressors come back into play. She should look at having some long periods of leave to try and recover properly from this experience for her own well being.

Residual Burnout

Long time expert on burnout, Dr. Geri Puleo believes it can take anything up to two years to fully recover from burnout and before this time, you could be vulnerable to residual burnout. For example, you might have left a job that has burned you out, had a few months rest and then gone back to work for a new company ready for a fresh start thinking you have recovered. She believes if in this time you fall back into your old familiar destructive habits you can crash quickly back into burnout...

She goes on to say that any triggers from your burnout that come to you in your new role may cause you to feel the same effects very quickly.

In the next chapter we will look at some of the other compounding effects COVID 19 has had on burnout...

Chapter Four - The COVID-19 Effect on Burnout

"**L**ife without experiences and sufferings is not life"-Socrates

I know we are all starting to become sick of hearing about the pandemic including myself and just want to move on with our lives, however it is important to understand how it has contributed to burnout over the past few years.

2020, saw a rapid rise in the already numbers of employees suffering burnout and I don't think it is going to end anytime soon. I think we can all agree that we had heard of burnout pre-twenty-twenty and some of us had experienced it.

Undeniably the increase in burnout in today's society has to be linked to the contribution of the stresses of the Global Pandemic and the ongoing aftermath of this virus today. We have all heard of the Great resignation and how businesses are struggling to recruit employees.

I have already touched briefly on the pandemic in chapter two however in this chapter I am going to discuss the social situations which occurred, which could have caused this increase in burnout cases.

People are re assessing their lives and taking breaks from everyday stress now more than ever. As a reminder, burnout tends to happen as people perceive there to be no resolution to their work stressors and that no one is listening to them. They may also have other issues going on either personally or in work ie: bullying at work or relationship issues at home which could be exacerbating these scenarios.

Pre pandemic, companies were all trying to run lean with supply chain and people, looking for efficiencies to keep those profits satisfactory. This was already putting pressure on workers in some areas, when the complexity of the pandemic came, suddenly there was no room for stretch to deal with the extra workload this brought with it, such as sickness and close contact leave. Consequently, this put more stress onto systems and people.

Life Changing effect of the Pandemic on People

Having someone die of COVID 19 has been a traumatic reality for millions of people word-wide. Some families losing multiple family members. In Western Australia we were lucky enough not to experience this phenomenon firsthand, unfortunately I did lose relatives and friends during this time in the UK which was devastating. We have all read stories or listened helplessly to the sad stories of face timing loved ones in ICU before ventilators were turned off, followed by lonely funerals.

I have nursing friends who were telling me the horror stories of shifts I could never have imagined in my career, with the losses of many and the stress of taking the virus home to loved ones.

Sadly, when the West Australian borders finally did open in mid-2022 one of my staff members, a nurse aged thirty-eight did catch covid and succumbed to it within weeks. It was devastating to think that we had been isolated for so long and the second it arrived in Western Australia it claimed him as a victim.

Like others who live in a different country to their parents and relatives, I lived with the stress of maybe never seeing family members again. I was ringing my parents daily for updates and begging them not to leave the house, even doing online shopping for them to stop them exposing themselves to the virus which was rampant in the UK at the time.

I can only imagine the stresses of the front line staff who were dealing with this time in epicenters of this pandemic. Including nursing homes, ambulance and hospital staff. The impact of this will be with them for a long time, manifesting in different ways.

Effects of Lock Downs on Health and Well Being

Without a vaccine, and seeing the chaos that was happening in Wuhan, northern Italy and Madrid, lock downs were the only responsible thing for governments to do at that time. Despite outcries from some people about our rights to freedom, most people understood that disease management rule number one is to isolate.

Governments did not want to lock down, the financial impact of doing so was immense on their countries' economies and some leaders held out as long as possible to try and prevent this.

It has been well documented since the pandemic that the countries that delayed their lock downs – such as the United Kingdom and United States – suffered more deaths and quicker spreads of infection in the early days of the pandemic than countries who pro-actively locked down quicker.

One of my managers, a young mother of three, told me that when we went into lock down in 2020, she loved the fact that all her children's extra activities, such as football and gymnastics, had been cancelled. Suddenly she and her husband enjoyed being at home with their children more. They had time to cook meals and sit at the table as a family, instead of having to grab takeaways on the way home from sports practices.

A lot of things went back to basics, jigsaws and board games sold out groups started on social media. Knitting and sewing became popular again; Karaoke and dancing lit up Tik Tok. Neighborhood Facebook groups became lifelines to people and there was an increase of pets being adopted.

As gyms closed and time outside was restricted, Peloton and other home fitness companies, share prices increased very quickly, the demand for home fitness equipment and lessons via the internet made new internet business models overnight.

On the flip side of this, sales of takeaway food and alcohol increased and a lot of people reported gaining weight, the consequences of alcoholism were also running high.

People were reluctant to go to hospital for fear of catching COVID and medical checkups were delayed. This unfortunately led to an increase in physical and mental illnesses going undiagnosed and untreated, as all resources were directed to COVID which was overwhelming hospitals.

On a recent trip to the UK I caught up with two friends who had each lost a parent during the pandemic. I was saddened to discover that both died from treatable cancers. Sadly I doubt these are isolated cases and the collateral damage from this pandemic will take years to research and collate.

My friend's father died from a naso-pharyngeal Non-Hodgkin's Lymphoma, My sister had suffered with this same cancer in 2018. She was able to have a course of eight chemotherapy sessions which put her into a remission. I could not help thinking how different her prognosis could have been if it had happened in 2020.

The world still had to go on functioning, we still needed food and essential supplies, and as a population we managed amazingly, given the circumstances and the tenacity and dedication of certain professions.

At the very beginning of countries' lock downs there was a massive mobilisation of technical equipment that was needed to enable this to happen. Most people that were not front line workers still needed to keep working from home.

I was communicating with an IT support worker in the finance sector, who had burned out twelve months into the pandemic in Sydney. He told me they had to purchase and install over two hundred computer set-ups in employees' home offices via video link and phone.

He and his team worked exhausting and stressful long hours, through weekends and evenings to enable company employees to function. We all know how frustrating it is to speak with an IT consultant when our PC goes wrong, and how frustrating it is for them when we do not understand what they are instructing us to do and how easily those instructions are lost in translation on a phone call. This man said even as he slept, he was dreaming he was on his phone helping frustrated employees overcome their IT issues.

He and some of his colleagues burned out very quickly during this time and he has since left his role. I do not believe this is an isolated incident for any front line service worker during this time, trying to pacify staff or customers whose business depends on them having online service and deliveries.

I heard from a work colleague about one Australian man, a CEO based in Hong Kong, who was isolated in his apartment during Hong Kong's long lock down. He was calling my colleague in Sydney during the night desperately contemplating suicide. He had not seen anyone for over twenty days and was desperate to get back to Australia and could not. Anyone who has lived in Hong Kong will know how strict their lock downs were and how small their apartments are.

Out of curiosity, I googled solitary confinement on Wikipedia: its states that it is a form of imprisonment in which the inmate lives in a single cell with little or no meaningful contact with other people. It goes on to say, it is used as a form of psychological torture and causes long-term negative physiological effects.

The United Nations general assembly Standard Minimum rules for treatment of prisoners were revised in 2015 to put restrictions on solitary confinement exceeding 15 days due to these negative effects...

Yet here we are locking people up in isolation in restricted spaces for months! The long term effects of this are yet to be fully realised.

During the pandemic lock downs, children were being educated remotely from home and isolated from their school friends. Expectant mothers were giving birth to their babies alone in hospital, nursing home residents were not allowed visits from their loved ones.

Tragically, the lock down itself provided the ideal situation for Gender based Violence and Child Abuse. Isolation with no escape or no one to report the situation to was one of the red flags for charities collaborating with vulnerable people.

Negativity and Stress Caused by Social Media.

For all the positives social media was providing to us over this time, there was also a dark side, there was a negativity that seemed to thrive in this time of tension and stress. It was a perfect storm, with populist political leaders making controversial claims of fake news about the pandemic and spamming up Twitter with late night unsubstantiated claims that were crashing the dollar.

From the birth of the Qanon website, taking people down the rabbit hole of conspiracy theories, such as the non-existence of the virus, then the virus being planted into face masks, to Bill Gates et al, conspiring to mass murder people with the vaccines, to reset the world and prevent global warming.

Once you fell down this search algorithm you were led to more and more outrageous conspiracies which fed into the minds of scared, vulnerable people looking for black and white answers to such complex issues.

Observing social media, you could sense by the dialogue on Facebook and Twitter, who was believing these by their posts. These political and social innuendos caused great stress to people on both sides who were trying to argue their point.

I remember having word from the UK that my granddaughter's granddad who had been in ICU in Colchester Hospital in Essex for eighteen days with COVID, was having the family visiting that day and I knew they were there to say their final goodbyes before his ventilator was switched off. He was 60 years old, worked full-time in sales and was the fourteenth person to die from Covid in that hospital, that week.

I was also on social media seeing people stating that the virus was a hoax. I was stressed and saddened to see how divisive the world was becoming while so many people were hurting.

The Effects of Working from Home on Health and Well-being

Doesn't working from home sound like a dream ? People who do not work from home, or are unable to work from home, think that people who do, have it easy and let's face it, in some ways they do! You don't have to think about what to wear. You do not have to sit in traffic for at least forty plus minutes a day and you can do your washing whenever you need to!

Unfortunately, there are downsides to working from home. Sue who worked in the financial sector, who's story I shared in chapter three, burned-out at home on two occasions during the lock downs in Sydney. Working in a high-stress area and having two teenage children at home doing Uni studies, she did not realise that the time she spent on her commute to and from work had allowed her to de-stress each way.

When she told me her story I suddenly realized that I used to do the same when I was flying! With my phone off I could either catch up on some work or watch a movie. When I stopped traveling in 2020 the boundaries between home and work no longer existed, as happened with many people.

Unfortunately, when working from home some people have struggled especially if you have a small home and don't have a dedicated place to work. I have spoken to friends who have had to work at a kitchen table with their husbands, trying to do meetings, take phone calls, and home schooling the children is challenging.

You also have the situation of people who live alone, and their work is their outlet and social life. Suddenly they are isolated by themselves for days on end without seeing anyone.

Working mothers have struggled to try and differentiate work and home time, especially when their children have been doing home schooling. This puts extra pressure and putting the children before their own work meaning they fall behind or have to work when their children have gone to bed.

Discussing all the above stressors that people have been facing since 2020, I believe we can safely associate the Pandemic as being a major cause of the ongoing stress we are all feeling and the increase in burnout in the current population.

Long COVID

I just want to spend a few minutes on the subject of 'Long COVID' or 'Post COVID condition' and discuss if this has had any impact on burnout. The symptoms of Long COVID can be very similar to burnout and to ME and other auto immune or post viral syndromes however it is currently too early to know why some people are more susceptible to this than others.

In August 2022, the UK attributed their low unemployment rates in part to Long COVID. The residual effect of this new phenomena could affect workforces around the world for years to come. Extensive studies are being carried out to look at the long-term effects of this virus.

Reading the current literature of which there is currently little, there seems to be two types of Post Covid conditions that are being identified by their symptoms.

The first is due to tissue damage to the lungs, heart muscle or other organs that can be identified however not treated which leaves patients with various levels of incapacitation. This is physical and can be diagnosed on scans and x rays.

The second type seems to be more idiopathic in nature with post viral symptoms such as fatigue and weakness, along with headaches, palpitations, and other symptoms such as brain fog and muscle aches. These symptoms are very common in other post viral illnesses and hard to diagnose and treat. The symptoms severity also does not seem to change in relation to the severity of which you suffered from the Covid virus itself.

A colleague I worked with is currently off with long COVID and is struggling to get back to work eight months post COVID, with her fatigue and headaches and was under a lot of pressure at work at the time of my burnout.

Does burnout make you more susceptible to long covid due to having a challenged immune system or are there a lot of people with undiagnosed long covid that is manifesting as Burnout?

For all I had been having burnout symptoms for over two years, my crash came as I was experiencing Covid symptoms, yet our borders were closed and I tested negative, yet I had lost my taste and smell and was sick for months. Did a post viral illness exacerbate my burnout or did my burnout exacerbate my viral illness?

Could this be one of the reasons for The Great Burnout? These are just questions I challenge myself with while writing.

I will just leave it there …

Chapter Five - Short and Long-term Symptoms of Burnout

" **N**ot all Storms come to Disrupt your Life, Some come to clear your Path" - Socrates

As excessive stress and fatigue build up over time, your body finds it difficult to regulate the stress hormones. Your blood pressure and heart rate become elevated, and your body remains in overdrive anticipating the next fight or flight episode. This then becomes an accumulative, perpetuating situation.

The physical and psychological symptoms below are the result of this status.

Short-Term Symptoms

- Loss of motivation
- Lack of energy to be productive
- Decreased satisfaction in your work.
- Procrastination
- Lack of concentration
- Irritability - Emotional outbursts at home and work
- Negativity
- Indigestion, Heartburn, or bowel problems.

- Jaw clenching or grinding your teeth while you are stressed or sleeping.
- Palpitations or fluttering in your chest.
- Exhaustion
- Insomnia
- Brain Fog

All of the above are related to high cortisol levels, sleep deprivation and fatigue and are the first signs of burnout. A break at this point should enable you to DE-stress, wind down and rest.

During this stage, symptoms on their own seem vague and you tend to think it's only a temporary thing, so you just try and 'work through it'. My advice is do not: Go and have a checkup with your doctor, try and take some stress leave, if you have adequate sick leave. Try to book a holiday – You need to change your mindset now – this is becoming an illness.

Prolonged stress associated with burnout causes the body's adrenal glands to release increased amounts of the stress hormone cortisol. Among other things cortisol is well known for causing 'post rush' hunger. How often do you hear people confess that they eat when under stress or they rush for the sweet stuff at 3pm afternoon tea time. Even if you aren't eating lots of sugar while stressed, cortisol slows down your metabolism, making it difficult for you to lose weight.

This constant cycle of stress can lead to insomnia or a disruption in your sleeping pattern. I used to go to sleep as soon as I was in bed, exhausted, then wake up around three or four am with a start, remembering something I hadn't done or needed to do.

I did not feel anxious when this happened and actually marveled at my brain's ability to remember these things whilst I was sleeping, reflecting back now, my mind was in overdrive and my body was not turning itself off completely while I slept.

It can be normal to wake up during the night, maybe more than once on occasions, however if this is outside of your normal routine and you have always been a good sleeper up until this point, it is abnormal to you. It is also definitely not normal to wake up during the night feeling anxious and having palpitations.

One of the things that helped me get back to sleep after these adrenaline rush wake ups, was having a meditation app on my phone. When I woke, I would put on my noise cancelling ear phones and listen to a meditation app, do the breathing exercises on it, which helped me to settle and sleep again. I would highly recommend this.

If you are relating to any of the above and connecting with this story, it's time to start planning some changes in your life. It is time to start managing your life and giving yourself some self-care.

The fight or flight mechanism our body uses to enable us to survive is only meant to be in short-term bursts. You will know from your own past experiences, when your body has exerted this mechanism to allow you to either run fast from a dangerous situation or cope with a stressful one, after it all settles down, when our body is calm again, we feel exhausted, we want to rest or sleep, to recover. This is our body's way of trying to claim back all the extra energy it has exerted.

Unfortunately, with burnout and other forms of chronic stress or anxiety, if you don't "blow off' these hormones in a fight or flight situations i.e. such as running, your body seems to eventually lose the ability to turn off these stress hormones. Consequently they are near constantly on high alert, meaning the slightest upset or stressor will trigger them as time goes by. Eventually this will start to affect the body's normal day-to-day functions both physically and mentally.

The time frame for the buildup of stress in the body is vague, as most people find it hard to pinpoint the actual time this stress began to creep into their work and personal lives. The physical and mental symptoms are discreet at first, becoming more noticeable as the burnout progresses.

How can you recognise these symptoms in the initial stages and distinguish them from exhaustion?

Like any other chronic illness, its about awareness. Once you know the symptoms you stop normalising them. Insomnia and indigestion are symptoms. Once you are aware of these symptoms you have to act.

You might start by feeling a 'bit of indigestion', suddenly you are buying bottles of antacid medications. You could be reaching for caffeine or sugary drinks at work to help boost you through the day.

Feeling exhausted during the day, if you are fit and healthy, is not normal, if you have no explanation for it: for example: Having young children who don't sleep and are keeping you awake. Long term exhaustion is a sign of something else going on with your body.

One thing which I did not even connect with my burnout at first was, about three years before my burnout, I started to suffer from unexplained toothache. It would come and go on its own and there was nothing wrong with my teeth.

That was until eventually, my back molars started to crack and break. Teeth grinding or bruxism is often related to stress and anxiety, unfortunately it was too late for me to prevent, and I still have to do jaw exercises to loosen up my jaw now, and I'm now the proud owner of eight crowns!

Long Term Symptoms

As with short term symptoms, there is no prescriptive time frame for the long-term symptoms of burnout, and every individual is unique, with different predisposing conditions, such as genetic and lifestyle factors. If you do have a family history of any of the long-term conditions, you will be more at risk of experiencing them yourself as time goes on.

Possible long-term effects of burnout include:

- Heart disease
- Type 2 diabetes
- Anxiety and depression
- Alcohol and substance misuse
- High blood pressure
- Inability to fight off infections, depleted immune system, causing complications to other co-morbidities.

Already at this point your body is inflamed, meaning you are subjecting it to excessive oxidative stress and damaging free radicals that are associated with cancer and atherosclerosis.

Oxidative Stress

Prolonged stress has been identified for a number of years now, as being one of multiple causes of oxidative stress. Simplistically described, oxidative stress, is caused by an imbalance between the production and accumulation of oxygen in your cells and tissue, which eventually leads to cell damage. It is being linked to numerous conditions including cancer.

Where you might relate to oxidative stress is reading about the effects of Anti-oxidants on your body. These are what help alleviate oxidative stress, however can't fight it other own. One way to check how inflamed you are is to ask your doctor to add a C-Reactive Protein (CRP) test onto your next routine blood test.

Predisposal to illnesses including viruses and infections:

This on its own can open a large pool of complications including

Guillaine Barr Syndrome (a severe complication of the influenza virus) and Epstein Barr (The common cold virus which has been linked to Multiple -Sclerosis).

At this point if you are still worrying about getting that pay rise or bonus, think very carefully. We had a profound saying when I was nursing: 'shrouds don't have pockets'. Stop worrying about letting anyone down – you will be replaced, they will survive. The question is, will you?

In the past, working as a nurse in a busy city coronary care unit, I witnesses patients,(predominantly men) admitted with chest pain and not willing to put their phones or laptops down while we tried to diagnose them. They were impatient to have us leave the room so they could take that last phone call or send that urgent email first. I've also seen them die there – not very often these days due to medications and interventional cardiology such as stents and implantable defibrillators, but they still do.

Type A and B personality Types:

In the 1950's two cardiologists (Friedman and Roseman) devised a psychological questionnaire which they believed identified what they called Pattern A and Pattern B personality traits.

Pattern A was the 'coronary prone behavior pattern', leading to detrimental physiological consequences to the heart. Pattern B was named the non-coronary prone pattern.

They stumbled across this phenomenon, by accident, due to a hospital upholsterer observing how in the cardiac waiting area chairs were wearing out considerably quicker, than in other waiting areas in the hospital.

Their questions were structured such as - Do You feel guilty if you use spare time to relax? And do you generally, move, walk, and eat rapidly? The subjects who answered yes to these types of questions were generally labeled as Type A and ones who answered No were labeled as Type B. They found most of their cardiology patients were Type A personalities. This lead on to more studies over the years associated with stress and blood serum levels such as cholesterol levels.

These behaviour patterns were eventually labeled Type A and Type B personalities and were fundamental in the ongoing study of psychological behaviour.

The reason I have mentioned type A&B personalities above is, being a Type A personality is also a risk factor for burnout. Type A personalities tend to be your hyper focused, high-energy people, always having new projects on the go. The ones who skydive and ski in their spare time. They tend to be high energy, competitive and can be your star employees. This is not what I had expected to find out when I was investigating burnout.

Sleep

I don't really cover sleep in great detail in this book, however research is demonstrating undeniably that healthy sleep is fundamental to good mental health.

I was once in a lecture with a sleep specialist who asked everyone in the room to raise their hand if they fell asleep at night within five minutes of putting their head on the pillow.

I was one of those people who proudly raised my hand, as she then went on to tell us that all of us who raised our hands were sleep deprived, which shocked me at the time.

Long-term sleep deprivation leads to irritability and can in extreme cases lead to psychosis. Long-term sleep dysfunction and insomnia are proven causes of mental health problems, medication dependency and even suicide.

Sleep is a whole complex subject on its own, so I am not going to delve any deeper into it, other than to say, if you are suffering from sleep problems, I would suggest before you start taking any medications, ask your doctor to request a sleep study for you.

How many times do you read about the corporate banker burning out, quitting, and buying a coffee shop? Or a hobby farm? These are the ones reassessing their lives, they never return to their old corporate life.

In leadership we have a duty of care to our employees to recognize the signs of burnout (as they may not themselves) and support them through this state. We should also be creating a culture that enables them to feel free to disclose burnout to us without feeling inadequate.

I did not feel comfortable enough to do this. My manager recognised I was exhausted however , so was he and there was no budget for extra manpower. I also did not have the insight to recognise my own symptoms fully, to know that I was about to crash and burn.

Self-help groups for burnout sufferers can be helpful, on the condition however I believe only if you are removed from the stressful situation first, you cannot fully switch off and start your journey to recovery, until this happens.

Imagine trying to cure a person from Post Traumatic Stress disorder and then putting them back into the same situation that caused it day after day.

As leaders, how do we recognise if our team is stressed and burned out?

Hindsight is a wonderful thing. In a conversation once with one of my employees, he confessed to feeling so tired, and told me that he was waking every morning at 4 am. With all my ignorance at the time, I told him I was doing the same, and suggested he maybe used the time to his advantage to catch up on some work!

OMG! I feel so ashamed of this now, I recommended this as it was what I was doing at the time!

Now, with my new found knowledge, I would see this immediately as a red flag ! Insomnia can be one of the first signs of burnout or stress. I would be starting to probe a bit more into his home life to see if all was OK.

If you are waking at 4 am every day and it is not your regular routine, then you are losing 2.5 hours of sleep per night. This is substantial, and it must be caught up with early nights or you are going to be sleep deprived over time.

Incidentally I found out at a later date my employee was going through a marriage breakup, if I had more insight at the time, I would have found this out !

Listen for the cues in meetings and one to ones, they will be there...

In my next chapter I will discuss the impact of burnout to companies and to the economy.

Chapter Six - The Impact of Burnout to Companies and the Economy

"The greatest lesson I have learned in life is that I still have a lot to learn" - **Socrates.'**

As the world is trying to 'live with COVID', and more people are resigning from their jobs and reassessing their quality of life. Manpower is in short supply, and we are hearing a new phrase, 'The Great Resignation'.

Emma Capper, a UK Wellbeing leader, wrote an article For HR News UK, after New Zealand's Prime minister's surprise announcement that she was stepping down from her role as she no longer had 'enough in the tank" to do her job.

She stated that's "Jacinda Ardern's resignation is a reflection of our time, but you don't need to be in a high-profile role to have been affected by the job. The pandemic years raised stress levels for many people and now the cost-of-living crisis is adding additional pressure.

She goes on to say employee burnout is a real concern for organisations also struggling because of the economic environment. However having a workforce that is physically and mentally well is essential for a company's performance.

My own thoughts on this are, long term, workers are burning out quicker than they can be replenished, from C suite executives to care workers. This is creating a perpetual revolving door situation for organisations and managers. Staff who are remaining in employment are picking up the slack for their co-workers who are either off sick or have resigned.

New employees are recruited and trained and regrettably don't stay once they recognize the dire situation of the job. Those who are being left behind are keeping the wheels turning working overtime and long hours in sometimes stressful situations.

As this situation continues, these employees start to get sick, they can't take leave so they either burn out or quietly quit as they can't see an end to the situation and feel they are not being listened to.

This shortage of employees can lead to competition for salaries and staff going to the highest payer, which then puts companies who are already juggling their budgets due to rising costs of products and under more pressure to balance budgets with rising costs of not just workforce competition. There is also the issue of rising and inefficient supply chain costs and inconveniences. This all contributes to high inflation, and, eventually, recession.

Every day we are seeing ambulances ramping at hospitals, queues in airports and supermarket shelves half empty. We are facing a world trying desperately to get back to normal, trying to ignore a virus which is still killing more people monthly at the time of writing this than any big flu epidemic, and is showing no signs of leaving us in peace anytime soon.

Pre-pandemic if you had a cold, you would come to work and sit at your desk buried in a pile of paper tissues. It is now no longer tolerated for people to come to work with a cough or cold anymore, so we have excess sickness due to COVID in its current – less severe, yet highly contagious form. We are also more susceptible to a multitude of other infections, having been isolated for so long from the outside world.

Lock downs have taken a huge psychological and physical toll on a lot of us, weight gain and alcohol being two side effects that affect our health and wellbeing substantially. People have faced their mortality, and some have had enough and decided life is too short and are leaving the workforce for good.

Burnout used to be called the carers' disease, unfortunately now it is appearing in professions that have never experienced it before.

Aging population

As populations are aging, workers are not only looking after their own children, some are also having to care for their aging family members as well. The last of the baby boomers are coming up to retirement age and are starting to need extra care in their elderly years.

When I began my nursing career in the 1980's the average age of a nurse was twenty-three. This has been growing since that time. I am aware of nurses in their seventies who are still working, a lot of them not through choice but necessity.

On a recent visit to the United Kingdom, I caught up with a friend who I trained had trained with as a nurse, who is still working. I was flabbergasted to hear how she had been a ward sister for many years however she now confessed to hating her job. She had downgraded voluntarily from her position and was now only doing a few days a week out of pity for the ward she was based on and was preparing this year to leave completely, saying she had had enough at fifty eight.

You cannot simply replace forty years of experience. Moving into the next ten years we are losing the last of the baby boomers from the workforce, the population is ageing and there are not enough of the next generation to be looking after them in their seventies, eighties and further.

We are looking over a cliff edge...

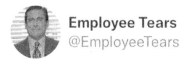

Employee Tears
@EmployeeTears

My job does this really cool thing where instead of hiring people to take on new roles in the company, they just add the extra workload to everyone else's job roles instead.

10:51 AM · 3/6/23

The Cost of Recruitment and On boarding

Working as a manager with profit & loss responsibility, I understand the fiscal cost of losing and replacing staff members. Any employee leaving their position creates a huge cost outlay to recruit and retrain to the level of the experienced employee you have just lost, counting in overtime to back fill for this permanent employee and supernumerary time to bring them up to competency level is huge.

Losing employees creates a gap in the workforce for up to six months, until the new employee is trained and competent in their role, the more specialised the role is, the longer this time tends to be.

I know businesses must function within the budgets provided and we must commit to a reliable workforce, so how do we strike a balance and make a company attractive so that people want to work for them and stay with them long-term?

Culture is the only thing that can differentiate your brand from others as competition mounts in the employment market.

The Loss of work hours

Work hours lost due to COVID-related illness and other viruses that are hitting us now and are costing companies productivity and eating into profits. Airlines are having to cancel flights due to sickness of their pilots and cabin crew. Businesses are losing sales due to supply chain delays.

The Health and Safety Executive UK reported that 17 million working days were lost in the UK in 2021/22 due to stress, depression or anxiety, and accounted for 55% of all work-related health cases.

Richard Branson famously said 'Take care of your employees and they will take care of your business.' I think this applies now more than ever.

When my husband and I split up, in a country with no family members around us, I was working as a full-time registered nurse at one of the city's busiest hospitals. I rotated early shifts and lates shifts, then every four weeks I did a block of two weeks night duty.

Being single, I was suddenly only able to work early shifts as I had no childcare. I could not leave them alone overnight, and late shifts meant they would have to come home from school to an empty house. I was not home until after ten pm sometimes and had to head back out at seven am!

I could not afford to leave my job as I had taken over the mortgage alone, I was in a constant state of anxiety, begging my colleagues to change shifts. I used all my sick leave for my night shifts and then reached a state of panic. I was always looking at the roster trying to plan.

This extra stress impeded on my work and family life. I have great empathy for all the front-line workers who are either juggling with their spouses' jobs or are single parents.

Later in my career, managing nursing staff and women, I soon learned that if a child of one of my employees was sick, very often it would fall under the mother's responsibility to use their sick leave or holidays to care for them.

In my situation I was eventually hauled into the office and asked about my sick time, which I confessed was due to the current lack of support I had with my children. I asked if I could do just early shifts until my children were old enough for me to leave them. In no uncertain terms I was told this was not an option and unfair on other staff, who would have to pick up all the late shifts and nights duty. Reluctantly, I had to sort out alternative employment and left a team and job I loved.

Could the manager have managed this differently to retain me? My children are now grown up and I could have now been supporting the single parents from a new generation. An astute manager would be capitalizing on this situation now. Flexibility is the key to retaining employees.

Do hospitals need to look at providing their own childcare facilities like some corporate companies do?

A few years later I applied for a position with a pharmaceutical company. I was excited at the prospect of a fully maintained company car, reasonable and flexible working hours, and no shift work. This seemed to be the way forward.

I was shortlisted for the position and was ecstatic to say the least. The last hurdle was to meet the managing director for his final tick of approval.

The year was 1999, he sat me down with a coffee for an 'informal' chat. After about 15 minutes of discussing the responsibility of the role and expectation he said to me: "I know you are a single parent, and I am taking a chance on you with this role. I do not ever want you to make me regret this." I was so grateful to be given the role, I made a promise not to let him down!

I never did let him or the company down. Quite to the contrary, I made sure I was on top of my game constantly. The people I feel I did let down though were my children, who were teenagers at the time and needed more time than I could give to them.

I am telling you this about myself to give you an understanding of why I believe I put my work first. This now fills me with so much regret, as I could never let the company know anything was wrong in my private life.

I believe I have carried this on through my career, to the benefit of my professional life unfortunately to the detriment of my long-term partner and my children.

Things have moved forward since then. Men are now allowed parental leave, Domestic violence leave is now given, which is amazing, as I remember having an employee once working for me from a safe house after escaping her husband who had kept her and her children captive in their home for two days.

No-one should be frightened of mentioning their marital status when they apply for a job. I still meet people too afraid to disclose their personal stress and anxiety in case they are seen as incompetent or not capable of a promotion.

I have witnessed an employee 'managed out' of a position due to his depression and anxiety and he later took his own life.

Companies seem to think because they subscribe to Employee Assistance Programs it is a tick box to creating a caring culture. It is just the first step, and the culture needs to come from the top.

Going back to cost the of burnout, my take is, we need to look after and nurture our employees over the next few years, the landscape has changed and we are all more fragile than ever post pandemic. Company culture and employment stability can have a huge impact on their bottom-line profits.

In the next chapter we will look at how managers can help navigate their employees through burnout and how friends, family and work colleagues can support someone with burnout.

Chapter Seven - How to Navigate Employees-Colleagues through Burnout

"T he secret of change is to focus all of your energy, not on fighting the old, but on building the new" - **Socrates**

If you have made it to this chapter, thank you so much for investing your time! How to navigate an employee or friend through burnout is something I have been asked on numerous occasions. Managers or colleagues suspect their colleague is struggling however do not know how to navigate or action it. I hope this chapter helps answer some to these issues, however I do not profess to have all the answers...

Whether you are a leader aiming to improve your leadership skills, with management and prevention of staff burnout or you're someone in the first stages of burnout contemplating whether you truly have it and don't know what to do about it, I am hoping this chapter will be of assistance.

To Employers, Human Resource Managers, Company CEO's.

If you are in a leadership role, and you have concern for an employee, it is critical if you want to keep your team member, to act early. This advice may go against what you really want to do as you are short staffed, busy, and short of resources.

None of this is important: in the long game you will lose them if you are not proactive, so take heed! The longer burnout is left untreated the longer it will take to recover from.

An article in the Harvard Business Review in 2017 titled Employee Burnout is a Problem with the Company not the Person; states that it is common for companies to treat burnout as a talent management or personal issue rather than a broader, organisational, challenge.

In earlier chapters I explained that burnout is not something that suddenly happens. Do not worry about a short bout of 'busyness': high-functioning teams with supportive managers can cope with the short-term stress, IF it has an end date and the employee is aware that there will be some down time at completion.

Subtle signs you are looking for are:

- Long-term unrelenting work hours with no end in sight.
- Changes to work routines that are out of the employee's control.

For example:

- picking up work and filling in for lost employees who have not been replaced.
- A company restructure that puts extra pressure on your employee.
- New systems, paperwork or software to use, without adequate support.
- Delays in external deliveries, outside of the employees control. IE: Awaiting, New PC, software or phone or the on boarding of a new employee - that is affecting their workload and lifting frustration levels.

Extra psychological stress either personal or work related to deal with.

- going through a separation or divorce
- trouble with children at home.

One alone of these touch points should not affect the employee to the point of burnout, it will be if there is two or more at play.

As a manager it is important to know what is going on with your teams. Use regular one-on-ones to try to gain more information about your team members. You can pick up cues if you are actively engaging with them.

One subtle sign in the first stage of burnout is the comment: "I'm just feeling exhausted all the time".

Do not miss this, it's an opportunity ... Ask them if they are sleeping well. If they say something like; "I have not been sleeping well lately", or "I keep waking up at 3 am", this is a chance for you to ask if there is anything on their minds and the big one - Is everything alright at home?

Their answer could be that they have a new puppy, but if they do tell you they are waking up thinking about work, take it on board.

In the past I have had employees with alcohol issues, children who are self-harming and domestic violence issues happening at home. All these things will impact on their work and up their risk factors to sickness, depression, and burnout.

As a manager, you need to make them take leave and use the employee assistance scheme if possible to facilitate them some counseling. Try to actively relieve some of their workload and stress. I will add at this point – Not to your own detriment as some of the managers mentioned in this book did this to their own detriment.

It is well documented that managers overload their competent staff as they believe they can cope with it, you can do this only up to a point, but beware. These are the ones who burn out.

If you can intervene at this exhausted stage, you are more likely to keep your staff member and they can get through this time. Otherwise, you notice they are starting to become negative in meetings, always putting the blockers on things and generally being cynical. Have a think about this, have they always been this way? If not, they are probably in the initial stages of burnout and need intervention immediately.

To Relatives, Spouses, Friends and Colleagues

If you are any of the above to someone who you suspect is burning out, support them, and listen to them. You probably know a lot more about their problems and personal life than their manager, so will pick up the signs and symptoms quicker. If someone is becoming cynical about their job or their company, they tend to still care about their role and have been passionate about it in the past and are hanging in there, hoping it's going to improve.

Persuade them to take time out, no excuses, explain about burnout and the consequences of not taking time out. Give them this book to read ! Awareness, like with any other illness or mental health issues is key. The three first line things you can persuade them to do are a doctor's check-up, stress leave and then a holiday!

Jen's Burnout

Jen was an active and conscientious nurse manager who took pride in the commitment she gave her job. She had worked in this position for over ten years without fault. She was high energy, physically fit and an 'attention to detail', perfectionist.

In 2018, her ward expanded in size, and she was given a 'promotion' with the extra responsibility of another area to manage including extra staff members reporting to her. This was a huge change management issue for both of her teams to integrate and adjust into.

When COVID arrived, she was exemplary with infection control. This was key to her patients whose immune systems were already compromised due to their chronic illness.

At the same time as her ward expansion and the recruiting of extra staff, her Human Resource department had a full turnover of staff and a new HR Software system was launched across the company for recruitment, which was not as agile as the original system, managers were used to using.

Sometimes through no fault of your own, outside influences can cause major roadblocks to your area of work and you have no way of controlling them. This is what happened here.

In this situation the total turnover of a company human resource team, as well as the introduction of a new software system contributed to a major failure in the support of the wards best interests and a ward manager's resignation due to burnout.

Nurses are renowned for changing their contracted hours. They tend to adjust to different situations in their lives and their families. Human resource teams need to be agile in changing contracts and salary levels, as well as recruiting new staff quickly, to keep the wards running effectively.

Unfortunately, in this case the entire process of recruitment change added extra complexities which slowed down recruitment to an unattainable pace. The result of this was that ideal candidates recruited by the manager were taking weeks to be onboarded, meaning the nurses took on positions in areas that were quicker to offer them new contracts.

Borders were closed and nurses were already in short supply, so this was a huge risk factor, yet no-one in HR seemed to be aware of the cliff the manager and her wards were just about to head over.

This caused great stress to Jen and her team. As shifts became shorter staffed, the nurses morale dropped on the ward and Jen became disheartened while repeatedly having to inform her staff there was no-one available to cover. She was working more and more shifts on the floor to fill in and support and was having to do her own role outside these hours.

As things became worse, she was coming in on her days off, could not take leave and was becoming increasingly frustrated at the system. Every time she highlighted the risk, she was told this was now the way and she would just have to learn to manage it.

One Monday morning after she had taken the weekend off, she returned to find a drug error had occurred, a staff member had administered medications to the wrong patient. The patient was fine however this incident had to be internally investigated and all staff on duty interviewed.

A Root Cause Analysis (RCA) was carried out by senior staff, this is an internal investigation which is carried out when errors occur.

This is a no blame investigation which encourages full disclosure and transparency, allowing lessons to be learned from the incidents and encourage reporting.

Despite this, it still had the effect of lowering staff morale even more and then there was a second incident...

Jen's direct manager was becoming really concerned about Jen's wellbeing at this point, as she was becoming very cynical and easily upset. After some discussions with the leadership team, it was agreed to close a few beds to deal with the short staffing and try to ease the pressure on her and her team to stabilise things, unfortunately nurses were starting to resign, and the effects of burnout were already started to affect Jen.

The following week she called her manager and said she had developed Shingles and handed over a sick note for one month off work.

Historically when Jen was off work, like a lot of other managers, she would still send some emails and text messages from her phone, this time her manager noticed there was radio silence from her and her phone was turned off the whole time.

I will say I believe this was good self-care by Jen at this point and she had recognised that she was sick and needed to take a break from all stress.

When people contract Shingles, their immune system tends to be at its lowest, and it can sometimes be stress that has taken them to this point. Her manager elevated her concerns about the HR issues sadly no-one seemed to be listening to the warning bells and they were dragging their heels to fix the issue.

Incidentally, I had shingles twice in the three years leading up to my resignation: one episode presented as chest pain and while I was in the emergency department the rash started to come out on my forehead.

Sadly, for the company and her colleagues, Jen returned to work and then handed in her resignation, stating she just needed time off, she had no more to give.

This is a classic summary of the impact of an internal problem upstream, caused due to departments working in silo's and a lack of communication and collaboration. If communication happens early in the concept stage with other departments, the blockers would have been identified before roll out and any issues could hopefully have been resolved then. Instead the impacts due to this were huge

- Staff frustration and stress
- Patient risk
- Loss of bed capacity, which would impact downstream onto other hospital wards and patients
- Loss of an experienced ward manager
- Loss of reputation of the ward culture which could impact further on recruitment.

In my next chapter I am going to discuss a worst case scenario of burnout, warning this could be a trigger.

Chapter Eight - The Relationship between Burnout, Depression and Anxiety

"**B**e Kind, for Everyone You Meet is Fighting a Hard Battle"-
Socrates

Whilst writing this book and having experienced burnout, I began to see certain similarities between burnout, anxiety and depression. They seemed to share certain features, could burnout be a predisposing factor to Anxiety and Depression in some cases?

Investigating further, there has been a significant number of studies delving into this, some conclusive to this being the case, some inconclusive other than the suspicion that there could be crossover.

High stress levels at work can be a factor in all three conditions. Interrupted sleep, cynicism and intrusive thoughts, exhaustion, withdrawing from social situations can all be signs of depression as well as burnout.

Palpitations, acute stress, lack of concentration and social anxiety can be signs of anxiety as well as burnout.

I found a study from 2019, 'The Relationship between Burnout, Depression and Anxiety: A systematic review and meta-analysis': it analysed all studies looking at this subject between 2007 and 2018, within its protocol.

Their findings revealed *no conclusive overlap between burnout and depression and burnout and anxiety, indicating that they are different and robust constructs. Future studies should focus on utilizing more longitudinal designs in order to assess the causal relationships between these variables.*

I would like to see more studies done post pandemic as all three of these conditions have been amplified over this time.

Self-Care, Step One

If you are an employee suspecting you have burnout, congratulations for having taken the initiative to read about it and if you have managed to read to this chapter you are still in the early stages of burnout and need to help yourself now... I mean immediately!

I know you will say you cannot because you are too busy and work can't do without you, the world will stop, and you are so indispensable. Well, if you are that indispensable you need to get off that merry-go-round now!

Take stress leave, even if it is just for a week to allow you to breath and take time to reflect and assess. This is good self-management: you are not weak, you are managing your health and need to do this so you can put things into perspective.

If you do not do this, it is self-abuse and you need to see someone to discuss why you are okay doing this to yourself.

Now, if you have come back from putting that leave in, I am now going to write something that is confronting and uncomfortable for me to write and for you to read.

I have put this in and taken it out so many times and regrettably I believe it needs a voice and it's important as a lesson not to have to learn yourself.

Johns Story

John (I have changed his name) was an employee of mine. He was mature, hardworking, and good with the customers. He came to me from a supervisory role with another company and said he just wanted to be one of the workers again; he did not need the stress.

I really liked him at interview and thought given time, he would be a talented team leader. After he had been with me around twelve months, I promoted him as manager for one of my teams. I now wonder if his 'downgrade', coming to work for us, as a front-line worker was due to stress or burnout with his previous company, however I don't know.

His team was customer service and patient focused and a very expert team. If we lost one of them, it took up to 12 months to have a new employee up to full competency level.

In 2008 after the Global Financial Crisis (G.F.C.), the company I worked for had a head freeze on all recruitment, and therefore half of his team who were being over worked to cover the shortfall, left to find roles with better staffing conditions (At the time I cursed them leaving, I now call this self-care and good management on their behalf!).

With his team being short staffed, John obviously went hands on tools to support them.

As the G.F.C. was hitting to deal with this the company restructured to a centralized management structure for Australia with the idea that they could centralize the resources and direct staff to where ever they were needed in the country.

At this point John stopped reporting to me and reported to a national manager based in Sydney. He started traveling there to management meetings and was also working a lot of weekends trying to assist his remaining team members, to prevent them leaving too.

I no longer had much contact with him however I had heard rumours he had started to become short-tempered, and it was thought he was drinking. He was clashing with his new manager and was not coping well with the new work structure. His colleagues were voicing their concerns about him not coping and he eventually went off on stress leave.

Just before he went on leave, his wife called me to see if there was anything I could do to change the structure and workload as she was becoming really concerned about his mental health.

Unfortunately there was nothing I could do however I did reached out to him and had a long chat over coffee about what was going on. He confided to me that as well as the pressures of the role, he was having trouble with his 24-year-old son who had become addicted to Methamphetamine and that he also hated the new company structure. Was he just cynical due to his burnout or was there genuine frustrations I am unsure.

Returning to work after three months' stress leave, there was no change in the staffing numbers of his team and the recruitment freeze was still in place. Despite all his best intentions, he could not cope: he was thought to be on anti-depressants and was drinking heavily.

From first-hand experience, his team was short-staffed and should have had one if not two extra heads on board. The personnel who left knew they weren't being listened to and knew when to move on; unfortunately this put more pressure on the ones who stayed.

Adding in the management complexity and his home stresses, sent this manager into a state of anxiety and depression. Which in my opinion now with retrospect, started as burnout. He had the work problems plus the added stress at home of his son's drug addiction.

After eventually going off on long-term sick leave due to his severe depression, John's employment was eventually terminated when it was realised he was not going to be able to return to work. Within twelve months he had taken his own life, he was fifty two.

Male suicide is on the rise and mental health is very complex, sadly John became collateral damage in a system that became broken and the extra stresses of his home life.

His suicide might have not been prevented in the bigger picture, however more due care and attention should be given to employees who are originally hardworking and passionate about their jobs. These people are the ones who end up either silently checking out, before eventually resigning or becoming cynical and clashing with management due to their frustrations. Often these employees become labeled as difficult.

I have just given you the most extreme case study and personal experience I have witnessed and if this has distressed you, apologies. It was an important example to give you and not to shy away from this. If it helps bring it home to someone how seriously a job can impact a person's life and save someone else from going through the same experience, I have succeeded by including it.

How Do We Break the Circuit and Prevent the Ongoing Journey to Burnout?

As discussed above, the only way to break the circuit is by someone recognising the signs and symptoms and acting on them.

As the individual running on that hamster wheel, you will not feel it coming on. It starts with a gradual decline, slowly going down that hill, increasing speed gradually, eventually leaving you in free fall.

It is a bit like growing old, it creeps in slowly. You do not notice it day by day and then suddenly you look back on photos and see the difference in your face and your body.

To You

- Are you constantly frustrated with your job?
- Are you becoming cynical of the company, your manager? Or your work colleagues?
- Do you feel like no-one is listening anymore to your frustrations?
- Look at your life, are things not going as planned?
- Are you exhausted and withdrawing from your social life?
- Are you no longer enjoying life and think about work even when you are not there?
- Are you feeling constantly exhausted, even after a good night's sleep?
- Do you wake up in the middle of the night thinking about work?
- Have you recently gone through a life-changing experience in your personal life?
- Are you not bouncing back quickly from colds and infections?

If you are answering yes to most of these questions, you are with no doubt suffering burnout. You need to dig deeper and ask yourself if you are experiencing these symptoms, what other symptoms are you experiencing?

Are you in good physical health and when was the last time you attended a health checkup or dental appointment?

Speak to family members about how you are going to approach this situation to make a change, as this is what is needed.

Can you speak to your employer and ask to reduce hours and take holidays or sick leave?

I know you think you are indispensable, but if you are experiencing more than two of these symptoms, you need to start making substantial changes to your lifestyle now.

If All Else Fails – Resign!

When I was dreaming of just sitting on the beach, and was planning my escape, I thought if all else failed and I could not afford to stay off work, I would sell my car and buy a camper van, rent my house out and just travel around Australia.

This is easier said than done! Go back to Maslow's theory and see how hard it is for most of us to do this.

I resigned three years previously from my position as I knew then things were not going to change, I was probably starting to experience the first stages of burnout at this point. I kept extending my notice as I didn't want to let anyone down and stupidly let my ego convince me no-one else could do my job. I eventually rescinded my notice and stayed.

Ironically if I had left my position then, I was in a position to have been able to apply for other jobs after a few weeks leave and would have had been back in the workforce. Remember the quicker you address this the quicker you will recover and can go back to the workforce.

Why is it that some people just resign and move on while others stay to the bitter end believing it will improve? Why don't they recognise their situation and prevent themselves reaching this stage of burnout?

Reasons tend to vary depending on their background and personal circumstances. For example, when victims of abusive relationships are asked why they did not leave sooner, they tend to say they believed things were going to get better.

For myself, with my work, I felt this way, I had always believed it was going to improve. Unfortunately, over the last few years, I was past the choice of moving on to another company, I was so exhausted physically and mentally I was unable to apply for other jobs, staying where I was for me was the place of least resistance. The idea of having to interview and start at another company was too exhausting to even think about.

I once attended a leadership meeting where employees were described in one of two categories. There were those who owned their jobs and those who rented them. This became a constant catchphrase across the leadership team I worked with at the time to describe an employee.

If they were renters they were there for money and they would leave for a better offer if it came up, to them the job was just functional. If they were an owner, they were committed and cared: it was more than just a job. In my opinion the latter would be the one who suffered burnout. I also believe I was an owner.

Have you ever been unhappy in a relationship and sat around for years in it trying to pluck up the courage to leave? You are entwined: joint bank accounts, children, pets, mortgages, security, friends... it's just too hard, for all you are not happy, its bearable so you stay.

Jobs can be the same: you're intertwined, your friends, work colleagues, your phone is the same, your pension, healthcare, salary, company car, laptop, it is all intertwined.

Have you ever left a relationship or a job and really regretted it? I will guarantee that 99% of you think no. You had no regrets and even think afterwards why I did not do it sooner. Our gut knows it's time for change, the universe is telling us it's time for change then life just plods on, and we choose to ignore the signs.

Our mind is talking us out of it, we tell ourselves it's going to get better but it's like groundhog day, it doesn't change and we sit in our little comfort zones getting our salaries at the end of the month...

Chapter Nine - Do More Women Burn out than Men?

"**A**ll *thinking Begins with Wondering"*-Socrates

Being an advocate of empowering women, and being from a generation, where we were told we could do it all, I found this a difficult one to write' the evidence is pointing to the fact that women are burning out at a higher rate than men.

McKinsey's report in September 2022 stated that 42% of women experienced burnout, in comparison to 35% of men.

A survey by Linked In revealed 74% of women are experiencing work place stress compared to 61% of men.

According to a recent report by McKinsey's on women in the workplace, the number one reason women are resigning or planning to resign from their positions is burnout. The survey goes on to report that 25% of women (compared to 21% of men) plan to quit their current job.

Putting my critical head on to the above results, and also trying not to be too pessimistic about them. We know that men do not like to disclose their thoughts and feelings, as some do not wish to be perceived as being weak.

Could this be a major factor in these numbers being higher in the female population? I am hoping this is the case, otherwise this will have a major impact on female leadership in coming years.

Carers of chronically ill people are recognised to suffer burnout; these also tend to be majority female. Females are also known for picking up most of the caring and domestic tasks at home as well as working fulltime. All these things will contribute to the higher burnout rates.

The AMA did a survey in late 2020 of 7,378 nurse respondents, 403 of these reported having experienced suicidal ideation within the past twelve months, which equals to 5.5% of the respondents. After conducting a multi variable analysis of the nurses data, researchers determined that burnout was strongly linked to suicidal ideation.

The nursing profession suffers a high incidence of burnout, especially since 2020. They are also seeing a high incidence of nurses leaving the profession due to this, which is not only sad but alarming, the pandemic has exacerbated this more in countries that were effected heavily by COVID.

When asking a friend of mine who is a nurse why she was leaving, she said she now felt like no-one cared or was listening to the staff at the 'coal face' and she could not see any improvements coming soon. She said she had no more to give and had also lost her mother during the pandemic and was re assessing her life.

New Zealand's prime minister Jacinda Ardern:

resigned in 2023 at the age of forty-two. Since being elected into office in 2017 she has been recognised as an inspirational figure to young women worldwide.

In 2019 she was tested by New Zealand's largest ever terrorist attack by a gunman, targeting a mosque in Christchurch with 51 fatalities. She was seen actively showing empathy and respect to the victims' families and her sympathy and involvement set an example to leaders and individuals worldwide and the respect and support of her countrymen.

She took on a second term of leadership in 2020, at a time of great worldwide turmoil, during the Covid-19 pandemic, having to make unpopular decisions that their government believed would be best for the country's health. New Zealand had been recognised as having one of the lowest death rates at the beginning of the pandemic due to their early proactive management but is suffering economically now.

During her time in leadership, she has also been pregnant and given birth to a daughter. She is only the second prime minister in history to have done so.

When I heard her resignation speech, my heart sank on hearing the words, nothing left in the tank to do it justice. I have heard these words so many times and when you hear them you know the person is suffering from burnout.

'My batteries are flat', 'I have nothing left to give'. 'There is nothing left in the tank': these are all words people with burnout used to describe how they feel. I was thinking about why they do this as I had done the same when I left my position.

In my opinion, and from my experience, you have dug so deep into those pockets of energy there is not one crumb left to pull you up, we are high energy people, we have used these resources so many times before and they have worked, all the resources are now gone. So you have the need to explain to people how bad this is, this is more than tiredness, more than exhaustion.

This is an emotional and physical emptiness, you are spent, which means you are unable to be confident you have the brainpower about the decisions you are making anymore.

Jacinda Ardern, left her position within two weeks of announcing her resignation and hopefully will make a full recovery and no doubt will see her in future in some inspirational role.

Can Women Have It All or Will They Burn Out Doing So?

Using Jacinda Ardern as an example, a young fit woman in the prime of her life, I have to ask this title question. Does her resignation reflect our current times? You also do not need to be in a high-profile role to have been affected by the challenges of a job. The pandemic years raised stress levels for most people and the cost-of-living crisis is now adding additional pressure.

Women in leadership experience high rates of burnout, exhaustion and chronic stress compared to men in similar positions. They are also more likely to work outside of work hours—in the evening and on a weekend.

HR News reports that burnout is hitting women in leadership roles the hardest, with at least 50% saying they are experiencing burnout at work. In 2020 in the UK alone a quarter of women in senior leadership roles said they wanted to downgrade their roles.

Christine's Story

Christine started with a corporate travel company in 2009 and managed a team of twelve women. She describes them collectively as the 'A' team, they worked hard, and they played hard. They were well paid and managed the travel companies largest corporate account in Australia and all the responsibilities that came with that.

She describes herself as a perfectionist by nature and liked to have control and get things done by whatever means. She feels now looking back, she may have 'set the bar' too high for her team and herself by always just dealing with things without complaining. Her team were paid large commissions; someone was always happy to do the extra work and get things done.

Around 2018, the ASX200 company they were contracted to for travel, started to hit pressures as China slowed down on demand for their product.

Christine was suddenly asked to start looking for efficiencies in her team. Her team she felt were already over stretched and were working to their full capacity, and she began to feel like she couldn't keep up with the work or the pressure that was being put on her.

At this point her and her partner had also decided they wanted to start a family and were going through IVF treatment which she also feels was stressful.

As the stress at work mounted and her days became longer, she said she could not be bothered cooking, so started picking up fast food on the way home from work. She confessed she was so exhausted some nights, when she came home, she couldn't be bothered to speak to her partner and would go straight to bed.

Christine said she had no problems sleeping throughout this whole experience, which was good, sadly, she had started to notice her hair falling out and she was experiencing abdominal bloating. On top of all this, she had not managed to get pregnant, and was starting to suffer from anxiety.

She became really worried about her health at this stage, however sadly could not afford to give up her job. She spoke to her partner about the worries she had about her health and wellbeing and felt he really wasn't listening to her. She mentioned going part time to him and he was not keen as he felt financially, they would not be able to manage.

One day driving home from work, when stopped at a red light, she started having palpitations, she said she felt her heart was pumping out of her chest and she thought she was going to have a heart attack, this experience really frightened her.

She went home and told her partner what had happened and they agreed she was now going part time, it was now non-negotiable.

As a manager she was not able to go part time on her pay level however there was a manager in another division who had been diagnosed with Crohn's disease and needed to reduce her hours as well.

The position was her original job, sharing the position they both worked three days a week and over lapped each other one day which meant they were both over everything that was happening, Christine believes this change saved her from burning out at this time. However she says for all she was part time, she was still no longer socializing; the thought of meeting friends socially gave her anxiety and if she did go out she felt like it was all too loud and would come home early.

The person she was job sharing with was also a successful manager and a perfectionist and they supported each other in this role however she felt the role was becoming less enjoyable as time went on with the client becoming more demanding and difficult.

Although things were better working less days, she said her team were working so hard and she confessed they all felt like ducks floating nicely on the surface, paddling like mad underneath the water.

In 2020 Christine says COVID was the straw that broke the camel's back! Her job changed completely overnight. As well as the change of working from home, she was dealing with company executives working for a multinational company, still needing to travel overseas, navigating closed borders and having to source visas and COVID information for each country that her clients were visiting. This information and rules changed erratically, and they were having to keep constantly up to date with this. Her email volume increased and the complaints from clients increased with all the travel frustrations.

Christine said one day when she was working from home, she just looked at all the emails she had and was overwhelmed. She says she switched off her computer and went to bed for the rest of the day and did not look at them again until the following morning and felt like she didn't care anymore.

Emails would become her big anxiety trigger. She could only read the first three lines of an email. She had brain fog and was struggling to concentrate on anything. She felt no-one in management was listening to them when they were telling them how busy and stressed they all were.

At this point, her job share partner was having flare ups of her Crohn's disease and Christine started to lose her hair again and was diagnosed with Alopecia.

In a desperate state, wrote a joint letter to their manager listing all their issues and what they felt needed to be done to fix the situation.

Christine and her work partner felt really optimistic after sending this letter, they felt it was well constructed and gave solutions to the issues and their manager, a woman, would be supportive as she was always advocating for female workers and held coffee morning talks on female empowerment.

Sadly, their manager did not even acknowledge the letter, after a few weeks they approached her, and she said in an offhand way she had forwarded it to her line manager.

This deflated them both and they knew there was no hope of change.

Her job share partner resigned and was not replaced and Christine carried on her three days a week and said she just 'turned up'. She was having to pick up the extra work, however she no longer cared, she says she cared about her team and their welfare but now no longer cared about the company or the client.

She started putting together an action plan to leave, she started a Pilates instructor course on her days off and decided she would like to make a lifestyle change. Once she finished her pilates course she resigned from the company after twelve years in employment. I asked how they reacted, and she said no-one really bothered.

I found this both depressing and concerning....

Christine is now working part time choosing her own hours as a Pilates and yoga instructor and is no longer experiencing symptoms of burnout, although confessed speaking to me and reflecting on it was triggering ...

In the next chapter I will discuss my own journey to recovery.

Chapter Ten - My Journey to Recovery

" If you can change your mindset, you can change your whole world"-Socrates

When discussing recovery in her TEDx webinar on burnout, Dr. Geri Puleo believes it takes around two years to fully recover from burnout. This resonates with me as even now, after eighteen months, if I become stressed or anxious over something, I become physically exhausted, and this can wipe me out for the day.

I have also become a huge procrastinator and must write myself lists to make myself do things, whereas when I was working, I was a very competent plate spinner. That was of course until eventually they all came crashing back down.

It is over eighteen months since my crash now and I still have the occasional episode of complete exhaustion where I am unable to build up the strength or energy to do anything for a couple of days. I try to just listen to my body over these times and go along with it and I recover and move on.

It tends to be after an extreme boost of exertion now this happens. For example, I over pushed my Pilates classes a few days in a row, added in a Christmas party late night and alcohol, and I feel as though I have gone backwards. This used to be effortlessly doable in my life before burnout, now I need to be aware and plan for these things or suffer the aftermath.

My only regrets now that I have left my company, are that I didn't recognise my burnout and do it earlier. Probably two years earlier and then I would not have left it to the latter stages of burnout. Regretfully, I did not do this, and now I have the honor of telling the story to you, which will hopefully help you or someone you know prevent it happening to them.

The good thing is most of the time, I can see my old self again and hope in the next few months to return to the workforce doing something I enjoy for an organisation that recognise the importance of a healthy culture and I will never let myself go down that toxic rabbit hole again.

Interesting the front-page story on Forbes Magazine for the first edition in 2023 'Is Health the New Company KPI!' It looks like hope could be out there. Thought leaders are now saying that burnout is the 'Canary in the Coalmine' with regards to a Company's health and culture, which I entirely agree with.

What was my recovery process and how did I get to where I am now?

The first four months I just rested, it was none negotiable, my body gave up, I had no choice in the matter. I was sick, I had infection after infection. I had been to my doctor during this time and had been given antibiotics and steroids for my chest and I had regular asthma checkups. After the antibiotics I would start with yeast infections and treatments for this, and the circle would continue.

After four months at home, I was starting to become troubled about my lack of improvement, so I went back to the doctors to voice this concern.

Socially I was doing nothing, if I did catch up with friends it was exhausting to listen and absorb conversations and even harder to speak, which was very unlike me. I was declining invitations, making up excuses not to attend; I just wanted to stay in my cave and not speak to anyone, the thought of getting ready and going out gave me anxiety.

I went to the doctor just before Christmas as I was really starting to worry about myself, I'd left my job four months previously and was expecting to be harvesting the fruits of my well-earned rest, yet instead I had turned into a hibernating elderly hermit. I was now convinced I had a terminal illness that was making me feel so exhausted and unable to think clearly. Probably some sort of blood cancer like leukemia was eating me away from within, attacking my bone marrow and killing me slowly. I was googling Motor Neuron disease and other neurological conditions, trying to come up with a diagnosis for why I felt this way.

It was helpful for me at this time to go and speak to a doctor and receive medical advice. I would advise anyone who is feeling this way not to ignore it, it is not a normal way to feel. Go and discuss your symptoms, have a full screening of blood tests performed and any other examination he or she suggests. A lot of diseases start with vague fatigues, such as diabetes and several types of cancer.

One of the blood tests he requested was a CRP (C Reactive Protein level). This is an indicator to detect inflammation in your body: it does not give you a cause or location but can motivate your doctor to investigate further.

My CRP was abnormally high, so my body was inflamed, which was probably predictable due to all the infections I had been having.

My iron and B12 levels were marginally low, I am vegetarian so this could be expected in my state of dietary neglect. On further reading vegetarian diets are frequently absent of Vitamin B12 and can be lacking in Omega 3 fatty acids, so I added in these daily supplements.

Due to feeling so exhausted and ill, I had fallen into a terrible habit of 'Uber Eating'. Whenever I felt hungry, and sometimes even when I did not ! I just opened my phone and looked through my favorite takeaways and pressed a button. Whether it was an Indian curries, pasta or pizza from a local Italian place, it was all so easy without much thought or energy. Thanks to COVID there was also doorstep dropping so you did not have to face the person for pleasantries who was delivering.

I could order these and even have the leftovers for breakfast or the following evening. I had started this habit after my partner had died the year before and we had gone into lock down. It started as a comfort eating thing living on my own and eventually became a necessity as I became sicker.

My C-Reactive Protein levels were a big concern for me, being highly inflamed translates to transmitting all sorts of free radicals and oxidative stress in the body. Inflammation is being identified more as being a risk factor for cancers and heart disease and other chronic illnesses. Knowing how bad this was for my health, it was scary as I was aware of how I felt so ill in myself. I had also gained a substantial amount of weight since I had left work due to my diet and lack of exercising.

After my blood results, I started trying to mindfully, making my own food, cutting down on the sugars and bad fats. I also started introducing more vegetables and fruit into my diet to boost my nutritional status.

For my anaemia, I commenced a three-month course of iron and vitamin B12 supplements which gradually improved my energy levels and I have continued taking these supplements since.

The only other thing I could do to increase my energy levels, as I was too weak to exercise, was to start losing some weight, which I knew should start to reduce inflammation and hopefully increase my energy.

I started to read about intermittent fasting as a way of doing this and really liked the idea.

I started this slowly at first, having nothing to eat after my evening meal around five and then delaying breakfast at first until ten am. This was challenging for the first few weeks as food was the first thing I thought about in the morning! Eating had become my go to comfort, and I had to break the habit.

After two weeks of leaving breakfast until ten, I pushed it to ten-thirty am and then every few days extended it by a further thirty minutes, reaching twelve-noon and then eventually two pm.

Instead of having carbs for my first meal, scrambled eggs, tomatoes and mushrooms became the new norm, when I extended it to later in the day, egg mayonnaise on crispbreads were enough to see me through to dinner.

For dinner I was having a salad with lots of seeds and nuts, avocado and roasted vegetables.

Once I was in this zone, I started to look further at my immunity, I had taken courses of antibiotics and steroids and wanted to improve my gut health, I started taking pre and probiotics before bed, this meant they had time to work during my fasting period.

To try and prevent any further chest infections or hair thinning, I commenced Zinc, vitamins C & D supplements.

Let us Talk Brain Fog

Until this point in my life, I had never really put much thought into my brain, it just worked and didn't really attract much attention.

The Cleveland Clinic website: describes brain fog as not a single definition or medical diagnosis, instead explains it as a cluster of cognitive symptoms that people experience including the following.

- Trouble focusing
- Difficulty staying attentive.
- Trouble remembering familiar details like names, places, and words.
- Slow reaction times and information processing.

- General fatigue and lethargy.
- Cloudiness of judgment
- Frequent loss of train of thought.

The way I have described it to people once I had crashed, it was all of the above and more. My brain was fried, this was no exaggeration, it was not just fried medium rare, it felt like a shriveled-up piece of black cinder still smoking, like a bush fire the day after it's been extinguished.

What I was experiencing is described in textbooks as brain fog, sadly for me this term is not a graphic enough description for how it felt.

I had always been sharp, full of spark with ideas flashing in and out of my head constantly. Now I was not just fogged up; my brain had left the room! Putting a conversation together left me exhausted and I struggled with my recall.

My concentration was zero and absorption of new information was practically nonexistent. This meant I just wanted to stay isolated from people and social situations as it was too much effort to even speak and listen.

I could not read or concentrate on the simplest of TV programs. I would sit staring at the television screen yet not absorb it. I spent hours just lying on the sofa in a state of enforced meditation.

At this point with retrospect, I recognise I was not keeping my body hydrated. I was eating high salt takeaway foods and mostly washing it down with tea and coffee with no extra intake of water.

I started adding in an Omega 3 supplement and Gingko Biloba* supplements to try and improve my brain function. If someone had recommended that Snake Oil would have helped me, I think I would have taken it at this time, I was so desperate to be back to normal. I have obviously improved since then, as I would not have been able to write this book twelve months ago.

By resting and letting my body recover at its own pace and not fighting it, I started with small steps doing daily walks. This was a huge challenge to me both psychologically and physically as I think my brain had started to convince me I could no longer do it.

On the flip side of this, I was also becoming really scared of what the consequences would be to me if I did not act on this now. I eventually committed myself to a slow long-haul approach.

After getting used to my daily dog walks I decided I needed something more, I joined a local hiking club and started doing a gentle hike once a week in the hills nearby which I had never in all my years in Perth discovered. I felt being out in nature and fresh air would do my body and mind good as well as learning about the local history. I knew no-one so did not have to speak much!

When I resigned from my position in the August, my plan was to have a few months off and return back to work after Christmas the following year fully refreshed. By February after six months off work I still did not feel ready to go back, so I decided to start a home renovation project that I had to cancel when my partner died, I did not think my roof would last another winter.

Just a small project – The replacement of my house roof, windows and all the weatherboards on the upper story. (I kid you not!).

After several expensive quotes to paint the weatherboards and window frames, I made the decision that as I was not working and had a limited budget, the least I could do was to paint the outside of the house myself during this process. After six months of lying on the sofa and gaining a lot of weight this wasn't a task for the faint hearted.

I started off painting the boards before they went up and after the first day, I ended up in bed for three days exhausted. After three days' rest, I started again and did another day, had two days off until eventually I was painting every day.

My office and laptop which I had an avoidance of during my burnout has now come back into my life and I am now writing a few hours a day.

I try to keep up my walking and have a new puppy which motivates me to do this, and I am hoping to drop at least another ten kilos so I can gain more energy.

I listened to my body and as soon as I had had enough, I stopped and rested. My son in law looked at me dubiously in those first few weeks and kept giving me details of other painters to contact and admitted to me later he never thought I would complete it.

I stuck at it reducing my recovery periods as I went, until I was skipping up the ladder on a morning. I kept up the intermittent fasting, going up on the ladder early in the morning as it was the height of summer in Perth and hot. I spent my days up on the scaffolding working on the opposite sides to the sun and giving my house a long awaited paint.

With all of this sunshine and exercise I was becoming physically healthy again. I loved sitting up there on the scaffolding just rolling that roller and paint brush, it felt therapeutic, and I didn't have to use my brain. Maybe I needed to become a manual worker as my brain was not functioning and I was starting to think maybe it was not coming back, this was the new norm for me.

Over two months I gave the house 3 coats of paint and lost twelve kilos in weight. I still could not read a book or watch anything complex on TV, but hey, I could move again, this was amazing.

I continued the supplements and the fasting from 6pm to 2pm and only ate two meals per day. I am now walking around twenty-two thousand steps a day with my dogs, and I try to do a few small hikes a month. Although I did get a bit adventurous on one hike and ended up burned again for about a week. This warned me that I needed still to be careful as I did not want to go back to where I was.

The dog walking is my salvation, as I am walking on the beach in the good weather and have a lovely lake nearby, I walk around in the winter. Note: when I was working there were some days, I struggled to do four thousand steps in a day, which proves how unhealthy I was.

A friend of mine loves meditation and goes away for weeks on end to meditate. She has desperately tried to convince me to take it up, I don't believe this is my thing, or would it be for a lot of people who are Type A personalities, regrettably we are probably the ones who need it !

As a compromise I do have a meditation App which I do put on if I am feeling extra stress or feel I need to rest and can't turn my mind off although I must confess I just tend to fall asleep while it's on. This still helps me with sleepless nights, so I am going to look into this more over time.

I now do Pilates three times a week, which I had to ease into slowly as after three sessions initially I was sick with a cold again and stop for a week. After another four sessions I finally caught COVID, which knocked me off my feet for three weeks.

I have discovered I go into everything with such zest and enthusiasm and then crash. I then have to patiently recover, easing in slowly, adding in recovery days, which I can gradually shorten the fitter I become.

I now no longer feel guilty doing nothing, I mentioned earlier in the book that I was creative, I am still struggling to find my creative streak, however, I have noticed now and again when its quiet and I'm resting, I am having ideas popping up in my head.

Let us talk about sleep!

Sleep hygiene to me is one of the most important things you can get right to improve your mental health. I watched my partner of seventeen years struggle with sleeping and the destruction on his mental health that this contributed to over time.

If you do feel your sleep hygiene is bad and you need help to sleep, the best advice I can give you is go and see a sleep specialist, have a sleep study carried out to ensure their is no obvious problem there that can be rectified such as Sleep Apnoea before you resort to to taking medications.

I no longer wake up during the night due to stress, if I did, I would put on the meditation app which would regulate my breathing and send me straight back off to sleep. I would highly recommend this to anyone who is suffering with broken sleep.

I do try to go to bed early now and if I have had a few late nights I try to make up the hours. Not having to think about work the following morning before going to sleep, helps. (except for drafting this book of course).

At least one night a week, I take myself off to my room, put on some music, shower, wash my hair, and have a pamper evening. I love this night and find it so beneficial. No screens just a bit of self-care before going to sleep early. All the above are part of my self-care and something that I had been neglecting for years to myself.

This experience although it has been a negative one has also allowed me space, I never thought I would have to self-reflect. Yes, I have gone a year and a half without a wage and lost out on all my pension contributions, however I feel like I have been given an opportunity to grow, change and to think independently again.

Sitting in my hairdressers eight months after commencing my new diet and supplements, I mention to her that my hair was snapping off at the front, I had a fringe about an inch long, right around my forehead which I had not cut in. She informed me it wasn't snapping off; it was new hair growth and asked me if I was taking any supplements, naming Zinc!

I have always been lucky enough to have had a lot of thick hair, but I had noticed the year before, my scalp was visible through my hair at the front. I had put this down to my age, I had obviously been so run down and depleted of nutrients that I had been losing my hair! It was wonderful to see the results of my new lifestyle and supplements paying off, with all this new hair growth.

The last supplement I added into my magic potion was magnesium, when your body is stressed, it burns through magnesium. Magnesium plays a key role in muscle and nerve cell function. Have you ever had an annoying intermittent twitch in your eye that no-one else can see but you think they can? It tends to come on when you have been stressed or tired.

Take a sachet of magnesium supplement and see how quickly it disappears. A colleague who I worked with was a naturopath and recommended this to me. Magnesium is also involved in energy production and can aid restful sleep. All the other supplements I took in the morning this one I took before bed with my pre and probiotics.

It's important to discuss with your doctor or pharmacist before commencing on any of these supplements if you have any other pre-existing conditions or medications that they could react with.

I also have no proof any of these supplements contributed to my healing other than the iron and B12.

As I mentioned earlier in this chapter, I do struggle with meditation however have found gentle exercise taking in my surroundings using all my senses, a helpful form of mindfulness. I also enjoy my relaxation sessions now at the end of Pilates my classes and would like to carry this on and look at doing some Yoga.

Hydration

Drinking water is not something we consciously think about, we just tend to drink when we are thirsty, however by the time our body lets us know we are thirsty we are already dehydrated.

We should be proactively drinking water throughout the day. The daily intake of water for a healthy person should be two to three litres depending on your body size, exercise, and dietary intake. In warmer weather you will need to increase this.

If you are burned out, you are probably not thinking about hydration and could be drinking more caffeine and sugary drinks to try and boost your energy levels.

Being dehydrated contributes to fatigue and feeling sluggish. Part of your rehabilitation should be to include plenty of water in your diet and trying to substitute soft drinks and coffee for water when possible.

Dietary Supplements I used to aid my recovery

Iron

Also found in: Red Meat, Dark Green Vegetables, peas, beans, lentils, nuts.

Properties - Red blood cell formation -Red Blood cells assist with transporting oxygen around the body. Deficiency causes tiredness & Lethargy as well as breathlessness and rapid heart beats

Vitamin B12

Also found in: Red Meat, including Liver and Kidneys which are a high source. Oily fish such as Sardines and Salmon, Eggs (Yolk). For Vegetarians Nutritional Yeast with added B12.

Properties - Needed for the formation of red blood cells and DNA. Essential for the development of the Brain & Nerve Cells.

Omega 3 Fatty Acids

Also found in: Oily fish, Flax seeds, Chia seeds, Hemp seeds, Walnuts & Edamame beans.

Properties - Fundamental to the development of cell membranes throughout the body and regulate blood clotting. It is an essential fatty acid and participates in multiple functions in the body. Associated with lowering levels of inflammation

Ginkgo Biloba

From; The Ginkgo Biloba Tree.

Properties -May promote blood circulation and possibly acts as an antioxidant to slow down changes in the brain. Commonly taken to assist memory and thought processes.

Magnesium

Also found in: Nuts especially almonds, green leafy vegetables, avocado, seeds, whole grains, milk, yoghurt.

Properties - Supports muscle and nerve function and energy production.

Zinc

Also found in: Red meat, poultry, fish, shellfish, eggs, some breakfast cereals, cow's milk, nuts & seeds, peas, beans & chickpeas, bread, cheese, and potatoes

(The body does not store excess Zinc so it must be constantly obtained).

Properties - Immune function, cell growth, wound healing, blood clotting, thyroid function.

Vitamin C

Also found in: Citrus fruits, kiwi, capsicum (bell peppers), green veg, tomatoes, strawberries.

Properties - Boosts immunity, wound healing, neutralizes free radicals. Assists with the development of several hormones and chemical messengers used in the brain and nervous system.

Vitamin D

Also found in: The main source comes from the action of sunlight on our skin. Only a small amount is absorbed from our diet.

- Fatty fish
- fish liver oils
- Beef liver
- egg yolks.

(Many people in colder climates will need to take supplements).

Properties - Critical in bone health, laboratory studies have shown it can reduce cancer cell growth, control infection, and reduce inflammation in the body.

Pre & Pro-biotics

Also found in: live yogurt, sauerkraut, whole grains, bananas, onions, garlic, soybeans.

Properties - Probiotics are living organisms (normal flora) that are beneficial to keeping your gut healthy. Prebiotics are foods to feed these human flora and encourage growth of them.

Note: This information is meant as a guide. It should not be used as personal medical advice without direction from a medical practitioner.

Other advice for ongoing Burnout

Once you have given your body time to rest, if you are feeling no better, it is important to seek medical advice and have screening done before you commence your journey to recovery. Ask for a blood screening to be done including Inflammatory markers.

Carry out the back log of screening appointments you have missed with your doctor and dentist, this is a start to good self-care and management.

When getting the results of your blood screening from your doctor ask him what supplements you should take to aid your recovery. If a doctor is not available a Naturopath or a Dietician can help with this.

.

Chapter Eleven - Future Proofing

"**P**refer Knowledge to Wealth, for one is transitory, the other is perpetual" - Socrates

Decision making

How do you look after your health by resigning, when you are committed to so much financially? Most people work full-time out of necessity; it is not often for pleasure. As our salaries increase, we tend to also upgrade our lives to our budget. We upgrade our houses, our cars, and our children's schools. We increase our spending accordingly and increase our credit card limits.

Suddenly you find yourself burned out with car and mortgage payments to meet, trapped in an impossible situation, unable to make any changes to your life for the sake of your health.

If you are really struggling and can't get time off work to recover and feel like you have no way out. Staying with your current company, you have to make changes and downgrade, if need be, to temporarily free yourself.

This is a hard decision for you, you have worked hard for everything you have earned and do not want to give it up. All I can advise you is, the longer you leave it the worse it is going to be to come back from.

The sooner you start to manage your situation, the sooner you are on the road to your recovery -act now!

You are no longer as effective at work now as you were, so you are already doing yourself an injustice. Depending on what you do for work, you are risking making major or minor errors. Mistakes and wrong decisions can cost you your job and your reputation.

For managers, it is hard for you to let someone take time off, however in the long run it is the best decision for all involved.

If you have sick leave, take it! I was good at giving this advice to my staff, I didn't divulge my own issues to my manager as he was new, and I was not fully aware of how bad my symptoms were or that I was going to crash like I did. I was also unaware of the long term health problems associated with burnout. After reading this book you are now educated to this and self-aware, you can no longer undo this knowledge.

When looking into decision making skills, to assist people with burnout, I started to read 'The Decision Book' which gives 50 models of strategic thinking.

I came across: The Consequences Model which I thought was appropriate. It states we often delay decisions because we have doubts, but, by not making that decision at the correct time is a decision in itself.

With this model Danish organisation theorist Kristian Kreiner and Soren Christianson encourage us to be courageous and make decisions on minimal information, IN TIME ...

Plan:

Start to put a plan in place as early as possible when you recognise your symptoms are probably burnout and are starting to affect your life either personally or at work.. Ask good friends and colleagues to give you an honest opinion of how they see you currently, they would have already noticed subtle changes in your behaviour.

Visit your doctor immediately and have a full check up to make sure firstly you are not suffering from some other underlying illness. Thyroid issues, anaemia or Type 2 diabetes, can make you very lethargic and affect your sleep.

Speak to your manager and confess to them what is going on. This can be very confronting and demoralizing for us, as we can feel like failures, You're Not!

Having doctors' advice or ongoing investigations can be powerful to help you back up that this is your health. You are actually managing your health! If you want to be a good leader you need to know how to manage yourself!

If you do not have sick leave, go to your bank and look at freezing loan repayments on your mortgage for a couple of months. It only takes two missed payments on a mortgage to attract default and credit ratings drop, this needs to be planned ahead so this doesn't happen.

If you recognize and manage this burnout early enough, three months off work should allow you to rest and recuperate at this stage.

I have a friend who has burned out and so decided to leave her job. She has sold her home in Sydney, put her possessions in storage, and is now just doing permanent house-sitting as she is not yet ready to go back to work. Not everyone is able to do this, if you have young children or pets its not an option, however if you are resourceful – you will think of a way! Before your brain fries...

The only final advice I can give you at this time is that you must think of this as an investment in yourself and your future – by allowing yourself this self-care and healing you can prevent complete burnout and the prospect of future health complications.

How to cope with burnout if you are still going to have to work?

So, you can't resign – the numbers don't add up. How then can you survive and get through this?

This is a difficult one for me to answer as I did not recognise the full extent of my burnout so did no self-management. Through the experience of writing this book however, I have learned some triggers and tip points along the way from people who have experienced it.

Firstly, it depends on what extent of fatigue you are experiencing. Bearing in mind a lot of this is not only down to hard work, but the stress of your job as well as maybe from the stresses you are experiencing at home. If none of this changes it is going to be difficult to keep working without experiencing burnout. (Do the same thing and get the same results).

Change needs to come from within you and how you manage yourself. We have already established that this can sometimes be a form of self-abuse. You have to finish all things and be all things to everyone. You believe you are indispensable and no-one can do the job like you, or you are frightened to take the time off in case someone else jumps into your position.

There needs to be a big change of mindset – a business coach or a counselor is worth investing in or even asking your company to invest in this for you, if you feel you have their support. If you don't trust yourself to make the correct decisions to put you first, then someone to bounce things off could be the answer.

Take regular holidays and while you are off make sure you have no contact with work. Exercise and practice some self-love such as remedial or relaxation massages and spas. Meditation is also beneficial if you are able to. This is essential for your health and well-being.

I do worry about people reading this who feel like there is no way out for them: for example, single parents who are sole caregivers and sole breadwinners on how they are going to cope? The answer has to be a change in job to something less stressful if nothing else is going to give I.e.: you have children with learning disabilities at home etc.

This is a really difficult one however I have to go back to total burnout and how hard that would be for you to deal with in the above situation. Burnout is physical, mental, and emotional exhaustion and you need to be able to address all three to recover.

One of my staff members who had gone through a bad divorce went away to a retreat for a week, where they were not allowed to speak for the whole time, just rest, meditate, yoga, walking and eating healthy foods. I remember when she told me about this, thinking how wonderful that would be – before I had burnout, I would have thought this as a form of torture now, of course I also told myself I was too busy to do it myself.

This is what self-management is about, recognising that you need to spend time on yourself, limit your workdays and hours and have regular breaks.

A day is twenty-four hours, divided into three eight-hour periods - eight to sleep, eight to work and eight for everything else you want to do. Obviously if you travel to work an hour each way that cuts into your own eight hours, still use it wisely - Podcast or meditation music, Audio books.

Delegate work, which I know can be almost impossible when staff numbers are low. I used to be frightened to overload anyone else as we were all suffering, by doing this, I overloaded myself.

If you refer back to most of the people who shared their story in this book they did the same. They tried to protect their staff and by doing so, overloaded themselves and they burned out.

One of the things I picked up on quickly as I became a manager was you can never say you are too busy ! Culturally it is not an option. You do what you need to do to get the work done, which means delegating it out. This culture is part of the issue of why we can't disclose burnout sometimes.

Burnout to stay at work:

Ask yourself the following questions to help you make an informed choice about what you should do.

1. Do you have personal issues outside of work that are contributing to your burnout? Yes / No
2. If Yes, are these personal issues permanent? Yes / No
3. Do you feel uncomfortable disclosing to your manager that you suspect you have burnout? Yes / No
4. Are you feeling overwhelmed with your workload or work/life balance? Yes / No
5. Do you have risk factors already associated with your health such as Diabetes or Heart problems? Yes / No
6. Are you overweight? Yes / No
7. Do you have heart disease or a strong family history of cardiovascular disease in the family? Yes / No
8. Are you experiencing sleep disturbances or lack of sleep ? Yes / No
9. Are you having feelings of your heart beating fast or fluttering in your chest ? Yes / No
10. Have you recently experienced breathlessness or hyperventilation? Yes/ No

If you have answered YES to more than two of the above questions you are probably experiencing signs of Burnout. Start making a plan to reduce your hours or change your job. This is an important warning, if you delay this decision you may end up suffering long term and have to take extended periods of leave to recover.

If you are answering YES to Questions 9 or 10 please seek medical attention immediately.

If you think you have burnout and want to make changes in your life answer the questions below:

1. Will your company allow you to take an extended period of leave to recover ? Yes / No
2. Would your company giving you extra support with a business coach or counselor to support you if you explained you needed support? Yes / No
3. Do you feel confident now you are aware of the symptoms of Burnout that you can manage yourself to claim back your energy and your health? Yes / No
4. Are you willing to make changes to your lifestyle at work and home to support your well being? Yes / No

If you are confidently answering YES to most of these questions you should be able to work through burnout back to health.

In chapter twelve we will look at what companies are doing now to prevent burnout...

Chapter Twelve - What are Companies Doing to Prevent Burnout

" **I** *cannot teach anybody anything, I can only make them think"* - *Socrates*

We currently have the perfect storm: The Great Resignation, The Great Burnout, an aging workforce, and a skill shortage worldwide.

How are companies addressing this to retain staff and assist keeping them healthy and well?

In 2017 Eric Garton wrote an article in the Harvard Business Review stating that the cost for the physical and psychological effects of burned-out employees in the US were estimated at $125 and $190 billion a year.

This estimate is measuring the tangible impacts of burnout, this does not include the intangible costs such as loss of productivity from employees with depleted energy who are quietly quitting in the background. People succumbing to long-term illnesses due to burnout such as depression, heart disease and other inflammatory diseases. These costing's were also calculated pre-pandemic, so will have increased exponentially since this time.

One of my old company CEO's in an opening speech at our Kick off conference stated that most employees when they were dissatisfied with their jobs, took up to two years to make the decision to move on. In those two years they became demotivated and their productivity slowed down. Their demotivation affected their whole team limiting beliefs and costing companies intangible amounts of money.

Having lived this experience, I know this to be true, this particular action is now referred to as quiet quitting and is now more prevalent than ever before.

Garton said that executives believe employee burnout as an individual issue rather than a broader organizational challenge. They tend to treat it as a talent management issue. He believes using workplace analytical tools to map employees' days can expose time spent in meetings and emails thus liberating an employee's day.

He believes this will give greater discipline to time management and free up the employee to do more productive things! I agree with all the above, it will help relieve stress in some cases. Email culture in particular can be out of control in some companies but mapping out employees days can be interpreted as micro management, which contributes to burnout.

By viewing burnout as a one-dimensional issue not a three dimen-sional one covering, work overload, personal life issues and stress, will not help individuals.

We need to examine what is going on in the background for the employee, what is demotivating them? What is causing them so much stress that they are burning out?

George Douros, in 2020, speaking on the subject of resilience training to prevent employee burnout, described burnout as 'the canary in the coal mine': *The solution is not stronger canaries.*

Being a coal miners' granddaughter I'm aware of the role of canaries in coal mines and find this statement very appropriate for Burnout. For those who are not familiar, the miners carried canaries in small cages with them basically as poisonous gas detectors , if the canary suddenly died, the miners knew there was gas present and it gave them time to escape. The canary responded to the effects of the gas sooner than the miner.

So, is it time to adopt staff well-being as a KPI? This is the title of an article of INTHEBLACK.CPA Australia (O'Connor T. Nov 2021) where she states that since COVID there is a new understanding that employee well-being is a critical factor influencing which organisations will survive our new uncertain normal and how many companies worldwide have made it their top concern.

She goes on to say, one way of capturing this is for companies to adopt a well-being key performance indicator, which is reported to the board based on the mental and physical health of their employees.

The workforce has lost a lot of female employees during the pandemic due to the extra pressure placed on them caring for aging parents, who have been taken out of or delayed from putting into nursing homes due to the pandemic, also managing sick children who are having an influx of illnesses post lock down.

Airlines are grappling to train up inexperienced staff and even the demand in passports has created mass recruitment and a demand on training up new personnel.

Alongside these mass recruitment's need to be robust human resource structures, also the awareness of the risk of burnout, to long-term staff that have been around throughout.

Being short staffed and then having the extra pressure of mentoring new staff into roles can be a stressful exhausting experience for these remaining staff members and it needs to be recognized and addressed.

Before looking at what companies are doing it is important to look at the way **Organizations Create Burnout.**

Dr. Geri Puleo in 2014 presented in one of her TEDx webinars a list of 10 Ways Organizations Create Burnout:

1.Poor Leadership

2.Lack of organizational caring

3.Role of other workers

4.Politics or sabotage

5.Lack of resources

6.Overemphasis on ROI (return on investment)

7.Work Overload *****

8.Poor Communication

9.Unethical or Illegal requirements

10.No Vision or Direction

Look at where work overload actually sits on the list ! We need to be critically examining the ones that come before work overload to gain a better understanding of burnout.

Companies must move from the age of efficiencies which tend to burn people out and resign to nurturing and managing their staff.

This is easier said than done, and the next few years are going to be a challenging time for companies, recruiting and retaining staff, meeting deadlines and financial targets. Stress creates stress, so if your manager is under pressure from above, he will project it down to his staff.

I wrote a post on Linked In, asking my contacts to tell me what their companies are doing to now prevent burnout. I only received one reply and it concerned meetings; there was nothing about self-care, hybrid working models or anything vaguely about employee well-being.

The only thing that separates good companies and good leaders is culture. People want to work in a positive environment. Looking into the future, the differentiation of culture in companies is going to be a standout for attracting and retaining talented staff.

We have people re-assessing their lives and lifestyles, we have lived more simple lives, buying less and socialising less during lock down. People have had more time to think and reflect on their lives and some have unfortunately had time to face their mortality.

We are seeing a bigger group of people moving out of cities into more rural areas for their health and lifestyle. House prices have increased dramatically during this time so cashing in on their equity has been a great advantage to many who lived in big cities.

Not everything is going back to normal. The thought and extra time needed for commuting back and forth to work has become an obstacle to some employees who no longer want to do the drives every day.

Employees do need to offer some flexibility if possible. Although think back to chapter three when I discussed Sue's burnout in the financial sector. She did not have set work hours so was working more, and found it exhausting trying to gauge the mood in meetings with no time to debrief with colleagues on the way in and out of them.

These are some of my own suggestions for retaining employees and keeping a happy workforce and a healthy culture.

Flexible Extra leave

- **Relocation Day** - IF you need to move house - one day a year maximum is allocated to do this. (This may not appear to be a big thing but with a rental crisis and moving house being classed as big personal stressors, having not to worry about a day off to move home can be a small thing a company could do to alleviate employee stress.)
- **Mental Health Day** - for the employee to do something for themselves
- **Children's sports days or grandparent days** - One day a year to allow you to attend your child or grandchild's concert or sporting event, I missed out on so many of these as a mother and the stress of watching the clock at work when you know your child is competing or performing is a feeling I know well.
- **Bereavement Leave or Special Care leave** - This should be individu-

ally negotiated it can be so personal.

When my partner died, one of the things I had to do was check my employment contract to see how many days leave I was entitled to and was so upset when I saw it was one day! Who on earth decided compassionate leave should be one day for a close family member?

I was lucky, I had sick leave I could take and did go to the doctors for a sick note in that first week, but I was shocked to think that in my time of grief, the company I had worked for had allocated this to me.

What if I had had no sick leave or annual leave to take at this devastating time. Companies need to really reassess this area to keep their employees healthy.

Three weeks should be mandatory for a close family member and maybe have accumulative days on top of this for service served. A person suffering this amount of grief should not be worrying about having to come to work as they cannot afford to stay away.

All of the above can make an employee feel like the company actually cares no matter how big it is.

Private Health Cover

One of the most fundamental things a company can do for their employees, no matter what country they live in, is provide private health cover for them and their family. I know some companies do this already; it's a small price to pay and means employees become more proactive with their own health, allowing health promotion and self-care to be more proactive by the employees.

You are not only allowing them access to a more flexible healthcare, but having assistance with important areas such as dentistry and physio means the company is pro actively keeping your employee and their family healthier and worry free.

This also allows employees to be seen and treated quicker aiding a quicker return to work.

Examples of this are knee and hip joint degeneration needing replacements, losing time off work due to incapacity. Females losing work due to suffering anaemia or pain whilst awaiting a hysterectomy.

Employee Well-being Manager

For larger companies as part of the Human Resource team, an Employee Well-being manager would be a great position to case manage staff members through burnout, health issues, workers comp, bullying, domestic violence, accidents, and rehabilitation.

Closely working with these employees on action plans of how to return to a healthy workplace. Most companies have the Employee Assistance Program, which is private and kept separate from the workplace and rightly so. This is good in some cases however there is no follow up with the employee.

Did it work? What else could we have done? Obviously this would have to be a voluntary thing the employer would divulge themselves is this needed more help and assistance.

The people I interviewed with burnout in the process of authoring this book, were very reluctant for me to use their names. They did not want to be identified by their employer or any future employer. They were scared this could go against them. This proves we are all talking about burnout yet we are still not recognising and accepting this as a genuine condition. The perception of it is that you are weak if you have suffered from it, not that you stayed around for too long in a bad culture doing the best you could.This has to change...

An employee well-being manager could bring this more to the forefront of the company to manage with a team approach.

Are employees taking their holidays, I know lots of employees who hoard their holidays in Australia, this is bad and also bad for a company's business, having to accrue for them.

The 4-day working week.

The four-day week, which is currently being trialed in the UK and in other countries with I believe some success. Here in Australia some private and govt organisations already offer 9-day fortnights, however only offered to approximately 30% of the working population.

Growing evidence is suggesting that reducing working hours, if done correctly, can be successful due to workers being more productive over the four days they are working.

These trials are ongoing but show that The Great Burnout is having an impact on the workforce and companies. It is fundamental to start exploring novel ways to resolve and future proof this issue.

Stop & Start

- **Stop** sending employees on time management courses if they complain their workloads are too much.
- **Start** recognising that burnout is a condition that is affecting them emotionally, physically, and mentally and will definitely affect productivity.
- **Stop** treating burnout as the individual's issue, it is the canary in the coalmine, a reflection on your business.
- **Stop** making it not okay to discuss burnout at work – its real and should not be a taboo subject that employees are frightened to confess to.
- **Stop** saying – 'She/He is just burned out' it is affecting your A team! Your diligent workers. Once they have reached a certain stage of

burnout you have lost them for good and their health is under threat. It's also a bit like spotting a mouse in your house... there is never just one mouse.

- **Start** trying to change the culture of the company if you are in a position to do so -If burnout has been part of your company's culture for a long period of time you will have employee burnout across multiple layers of the workforce.
- **Start** encouraging regular holidays – make them compulsory, they are necessary for prevention.
- **Start** encouraging normal working hours.
- **Stop** sending emails outside of work hours.
- **Stop** texting and calling staff outside of work hours.
- **Start** looking at your management structure, is micromanagement or bullying helping to burnout your employees.

In Chapter thirteen we will look at burnout prevention, to try and look at ways to help you recognise and work through burnout early. We will also look at people returning to work like myself to prevent residual burnout happening.

Chapter Thirteen - Prevention is Better than Cure

"*F*alling down is not a failure, failure comes when you stay where you have fallen" *Socrates*

I know this chapter probably feels like closing the door after the horse has bolted however even for myself as I am about to dip my toe back into the workforce again very soon, we need to Litmus check and be aware and prepared.

Most of us are tuned in to working hard and doing the best we can or we are ambitious to make it to the top. Whether you can see yourself going down the rabbit hole of burning yourself out or like myself wanting to make sure I see the warning signs this time. We must be aware that prevention is better than cure.

My partner, I believe could see what I was doing to myself, though he didn't want to stand in the way of my career.

A few years before I burned out, when I was feeling particularly frustrated about my role, he sent me a card with this poem inside. Re reading this now is so meaningful to me and I wished I had taken notice of it more at the time.

The Indispensable Man

Sometime when you're feeling important.
  Sometime when your ego's in bloom
  Sometime when you take it for granted.
  You're the best qualified in the room,

Sometime when you feel that you're going.
  Would leave an unfillable hole,
  Just follow these simple instructions
  And see how they humble your soul.

Take a bucket and fill it with water,
  Put your hand in it, up to the wrist,
  Pull it out and the hole that's remaining.
  Is a measure of how you will be missed.

You can splash all you wish when you enter,
  You may stir up the water galore,
  But stop and you will find in no time.
  It looks quite the same as before.

The Moral of this quaint example
  Is to do just the best that you can,
  Be proud of yourself but remember,
  There is no indispensable man.

British Poet - unknown.

I'm a great believer that burnout is multi-faceted. If your personal life is
going well and you are supported, you can handle your work life (unless

there are big stresses at work). If your work life is supported correctly, you can handle your personal life. The problem comes as in everyday life when the wheel falls off one aspect of your life, requiring extra emotional energy from you.

With myself I was dealing with mental illness in my family, and I was trying to be everything to everyone as well as being a manager to thirteen direct reports, who in turn had their issues.

I had gone from having a supportive partner who was always there for advice and support to a partner who was ill, suffering from anxiety and depression.

Suddenly guilt was always with me when I was working late and traveling. I no longer wanted to tell him my issues as he was then worrying and over thinking them too. So I kept them all to myself.

Listening to our bodies

This is so important and we need to get better at it! Not just for detecting burnout, also for all physical and mental issues. Our body is very good at giving us signals, we just need to get better at reading them. I have read so many cases of young people experiencing exhaustion and weakness and they have too late been diagnosed with stage 4, ovarian or bowel cancer for example.

If you are feeling abnormally fatigued for longer than a week you need to rest up and get checked. Are you getting sick as soon as you rest or go on leave? This is a sign that you have been working in stress for a prolonged period of time and when you eventually rest and your cortisol levels start to drop, leaving your body susceptible to infection.

Are you practicing self-care still? early nights, meditation or relaxation, healthy nutritious diet, exercise, and hydration?

These are a non-negotiable during this time ...

Listening to our minds:

Are you struggling to focus on things? Are you losing patience with situations or people. Are you overreacting to situations? These are all signs of burnout. Are you becoming distracted at work with personal things or distracted at home with work things?

Do you struggle to switch off work when you go on leave or even on the weekend?

Are your weekends no lonnger replenishing your energy? Stop! Take leave and rest.

Financial hand cuffs

How can we afford the breakout of them. I would ask – How can we not afford the breakout of them? You might think this is an easy answer however its simple – Shrouds don't have pockets!

How do we make the break ? - Negotiations with your current employer would be the first step, if you are wanting the security of staying with the company you work for in your current position. You are currently in a good position and if you are a valuable member of the team they will want to keep you long term.

Explaining face to face if possible, that you are in desperate need of a break and concerned that if you do not, you feel you could burn out. That you are worried about your health, giving symptoms if necessary.

If you do this face to face follow up with an email thanking your manager for taking you seriously and having this granted will allow you to come back refreshed.

Better still have a plan ready for how business will look in your absence, do you have someone who could step up for three or six months? If you don't work for a big organisation, it could be difficult for them to recruit to fill a position for three to six months and if your burnout is due mostly to the pressure and stress of your job then no doubt there will be multiple layers of burned out workers and managers around you.

If this is the case then you are going to have to assess whether you really want to stay there long term. If they refuse your request saying there is no way they can spare you for this time then you really need to think carefully about how you are going to handle this short and long term.

Are you listening to your Ego ?

Ego comes before a fall not pride...(I have made that up, but believe it) I know an employee, who was struggling with the stress of his management role and was offered a role one step below and he refused. . . six months later he crashed and left.

Some people won't take leave as they are scared someone will take over their role and in their absence do better than them ! This is classic and more common than you think. These are also classic signs of being sabotaged by your own ego. Is this the reason why you do not take holidays or are working long hours ?

Some managers have been known to use a competition tactics on employees to keep them 'on their toes' playing ego's games. Telling one employee that the other is doing a great job. Do not buy into this rhetoric, its destructive and a sign of poor work culture.

Start writing things down, sometime when you see the reasons why you won't take leave in writing, they will resonate more with you.

Residual Burnout

For myself and anyone else returning back to the workforce who has burned out in the past, you are more at risk of burning out again so must be more vigilant for the signs.

Recently whilst writing this book, I started to put myself under a bit of pressure to finish it and unbelievably started to go back to a few old habits.

I was writing for long periods and eating at my desk. I started waking up in the middle of the night stressing if this book was really any good. Impostor syndrome started to creep in - no one was going to buy it or like it so why was I bothering. Then I had to buy a bottle of Gaviscon for my heartburn and recognised where this was going.

So, I stopped, totally, took a few days off (I had been writing every day for weeks.) My eyes were dry and my wrists were aching. I reminded myself of the reason I was writing this book, to warn others of the dangers of burnout!

I started with the meditation music, took a few days off from writing and did more outdoor activities and pulled myself back into line.

I have the knowledge and I know how to manage it now and so do you now you have read my book...

Conclusion

There is no doubt in society today that the stresses of the pandemic have exacerbated burnout and it will continue to be a contributing factor impeding work forces over the next few years.

Early awareness and intervention in the first stages of burnout can help prevent total burnout and aid recovery. These factors need to be taken into consideration by companies for employee health and well-being programs.

Burnout should not be a taboo subject, it is not an individual issue, it is a company issue and should be treated as such. High level employees should not be stigmatised by staying on at a company to the point of burnout.

Burnout and employee well-being should be part of a company's KPI's as they reflect on a company's 'whole well-being'.

Total burnout can take up to two years to recover from and a slow, steady, holistic approach is the way to recovery.

More studies need to be carried out to better define burnout and allow it to be recognised better by the World Health Organization.

Epilogue

Thank you for staying with me to the end of The Great Burnout, I have found it therapeutic to write this journey and I am hoping you will find it of some assistance to your own journey.

I am now on the last few weeks of my leave and I am excited to be returning to the workforce with a new refreshed energy.

Bringing this book to a close, I am seeing burnout becoming a topical media headline and I am hoping my experience and the experiences of the people who kindly let me tell their stories are of assistance.

Please look after yourselves people and remember we are all only humans doing the best we can.

Finally - Did I go and sit on the beach ? HELL YES! I did lots especially with my dogs and after my Pilates classes, when I would swim in the sea....

Best wishes Julie x

If you would like to stay in touch and follow my journey, follow me on;

Instagram @non_fiction_novice or **Twitter** @nonfictionnovice

Acknowledgments

Trying to write a book about burnout when I was suffering from burnout was a challenge but a story I needed to tell. I know when I first told friends I was planning on writing a book it was a bit like telling my son in law I was going to paint the outside of my house. No one actually said anything but their expressions told me their thoughts.

Thank you to all who have encouraged me, read and given me their opinions and thoughts and sent me articles during this time it's amazing to see the interest I've created.

Thanks to my granddaughter Isabella for her editing and corrections of my 'too English' grammar and my dogs for sitting in my study with me every day writing keeping me company.

To my family and friends who had faith in me and including the ones who are no longer here to see the final result...

Finally a big Thank you to my cousin Christine Todd and her husband Jean, both published authors for giving me the inspiration and encouragement to do so. RIP Jean you will be missed x

About the Author

J ulie Thompson was born in the Northeast of England. She emigrated to Perth when she was thirty as a registered nurse.

She has two grown up children and three grandchildren. She lives near the coast, twelve kilometres north of Perth, Western Australia with her two dogs and three cats.

References

BC News, U. S. (2023, February 19). *Jacinda Ardern, Resignation Speech BBC News, You Tube.* Retrieved from You Tube .com: http://www.YouTube.com

Berg. S, MS. (2022 May 17) AMA. Burnout Benchmark:28% unhappy with current healthcare job. https://www.ama-assn.org/practice-mana gement/physician-health/burnout-benchmoark-28-unhappy-current -health-care-job

Campbell F, (2022, September). *How to support employees with 'nothing left in the tank.* Retrieved from HR News: https://hrnews.co.uk/burnout-how-to-support-employees-with-nothing-left-in-the-tank/

Capper, E . (2023, January 27). *HR news.* Retrieved from hrnews.co.uk: https://hrnews.co.uk/burnout-how-to-support-employees-with-not hing-left-in-the-tank/

Chan, T. (2020, March). *The Nutrition Source - Vit C.* Retrieved from hsph.harvard: Https://www.hsph.harvard.edu/nutritionsource/vitamin-C

Creed, R. (2020,November 5) Gazette Standard-*Colchester Hospital records 14 covid deaths in one week.* https:/www.gazette-news.co.uk/new s/18846721.colchester-hospital.records-14-covid-deaths-one-week/

Douros. G. (Jun 2020). Burnout is the Canary in the coalmine; the solution is not stronger canaries . *Emerg Med Australs 32(3)*, 518-519.

Employee Tears (2023,March 6) Instagram @EmployeesTears

Gartin,Eric. (2017, April 6th). *Employee Burnout is a Problem wiht the Company, Not the Person.* Retrieved from HBR.org: https://hbr.org/2017/ 04/employee-burnout-is-a-problem-with-the-company-not-the-pe rson#

Georganta, K. Montgomery, A. Panagiota, K. (March 13, 2019) The Relationship Between Burnout, Depression and Anxiety: A Systematic Review and Meta -Analysis. Front Psychology 10:284.doi:10.3389/fp-syg.2019.00284. eCollection 2019.

Kearns, A. M. (2022, April 16). *Adrenal Fatigue:what causes it?* Retrieved from mayo clinic.org: https://www.mayoclinic.org/diseases

Krogerus M, T. R. (2008). The Consequences Model. In K. M. R., *The Decision Book* (pp. 34,35). London: Profile books .

Lee. J. Dr. (n.d.). *AIA Think Well.* Retrieved from AIA.com.au: https://ww w.aia.com.au/en/individual/onelife/think-well/dr-jaime-lee-how-to-ask-for-a-mental-health-day.html

Loder. V . (2015, 01 30). *www.forbes.com how to prevent burnout.* Retrieved from https://www.forbes.com/sites/vanessaloder/2015/01/30 /how-to-prevent-burnout-13-signs-youre-on-the-edge

A.H., Maslow. (1943). A Theory of Human Motivation. *Psychological Review 504370,* 370-396.

McLeod, S. (2022, April 2022). *Simply Psychology.* Retrieved from Simply Psychology/maslow.html: https:/www.simplypsychology/maslow.html

N.K. (2023, February 2). *Wikipedia.* Retrieved from Wikipedia.org: https://en.wikipedia.org/wiki/Solitary_confinement

O'Connor,T. (2021, November 1st). *INTHEBLACK CPA Australia.* Retrieved from intheblack.CPAAustralia.com.au: https://intheblack.cpaaustralia.c omau/work-life/adopt-staff-wellbeing-as-a-kpi

Puleo, G. Dr. (2011). *Causes and Maintenance Factors of Employee Burnout During Transformational Organizational Change.* Retrieved 7 28, 2022, from http://gradworks.umi.com/34/75/3475108.html

Puleo G, Dr. (2014, February 26). *Burnout PTSD and ADAAA- New Way to Work.* Retrieved from Tedx: https://a-new-way-to-wor.com/2014/02/ 26/tedx-presentation-burnout,change,stress,working

Robinson, B.E. PHD (November 18,2020) The Surprising Difference Between Stress and Burnout

S.Schiavone, V. K.-H. (2013, March 14th). *Severe Life Stress & Oxidative Stress in the Brain: From ANimal Models to Human Pathology.* Retrieved from liebertpub.com: https://doi.org/10.1089/ars.2012.4720

Service, R. W. (2016, May 27). Be Master of your petty annoyances and conserve your energies for the big worthwhile things. *Quotationcelebration.wordpress.com.*

Socrates. (2022, July 2022). *"Socrates Quotes" Quoteslyfe.* Retrieved from quoteslyfe.com: <https://www.quoteslyfe.com/quote/My-friend-care-for-your-psycge-know-160421

Staff, M. C. (2021, june 5th). Retrieved from mayoclinic.org: https//ww w.mayoclinicorg/healthy-lifestyle/in-depth/burnout/art-20046642

(NK). T.H.Chan. *hsph.harvard.* Retrieved from The Nutrition Source - Zinc: Https:/www.hsph.harvard.edu/nutritionsource/Zinc

(NK). T.H. Chan. *The Nutrition Source - Magnesium.* Retrieved from hsph.harvard.edu: Https://www.hsph.harvard.edu/nutritionsource/-magnesium

(NK). T.H. Chan. *The Nutritional Source.* Retrieved from hsph.harvard.edu: https:/www.hsph.harvard.edu/nutritionsource/iron

(N.K) T.H.Chan (2022, November). *The Nutrition Source.* Retrieved from hsph.harvard.edu: Https://www.hsph.harvard.edu/nutritionsource/vitamin-d

Unknown Author (2022, June 14). *Strategies for Busting Up Brain Fog.* Retrieved from health.clevelandclinic.org: https:/health.clevelandclinic.org/bain-fog/amp/

Unknown Author (21/22). *https://www.hse.gov.uk/statistics/.* London : government website.

Vegetarian Society UK. (2023). *Vegetarian Society Info Hub.* Retrieved from Vegsoc.org: https://vegsoc.org/info-hub/health-and-nutrition/zinc/

World Health Organisation. (2019). Factors Influencing health status. *11th International Classification of Diseases.*